ADHD
2021

A Revolutionary New Approach to
ADD/ADHD

The information and advice presented in this book are not meant to substitute for the advice of your physician, your child's pediatrician, or other trained healthcare professionals. You are advised to consult with healthcare professionals with regard to all matters that may require medical attention or diagnosis and to check with a physician before administering or undertaking any course of treatment or making any significant changes to your child's diet.

The names and some identifying characteristics of some of the individuals presented in this book have been changed to protect their privacy. Any resulting resemblance to persons living or dead is entirely coincidental and unintentional.

Contents

Cover

Title Page

Copyright

Chapter 1: A Spectrum of Traits

Chapter 2: Understanding the Demon of the Mind

Chapter 3: The Cerebellum Connection

Chapter 4: The Healing Power of Connection

Chapter 5: Find Your Right Difficult

Chapter 6: Create Stellar Environments

Chapter 7: Move to Focus, Move to Motivate: The Power of Exercise

Chapter 8: Medication: The Most Powerful Tool Everyone Fears

Chapter 9: Putting It All Together: Find Your Feel and Make It Real

CHAPTER 1

|

A Spectrum of Traits

Who are we, the people who have ADHD?

We are the problem kid who drives his parents crazy by being totally disorganized, unable to follow through on anything, incapable of cleaning up a room, or washing dishes, or performing just about any assigned task; the one who is forever interrupting, making excuses for work not done, and generally functioning far below potential in most areas. We are the kid who gets daily lectures on how we're squandering our talent, wasting the golden opportunity that our innate ability gives us to do well, and failing to make good use of all that our parents have provided.

We are also sometimes the talented executive who keeps falling short due to missed deadlines, forgotten obligations, social faux pas, and blown opportunities. Too often we are the addicts, the misfits, the unemployed, and the criminals who are just one diagnosis and treatment plan away from turning it all around. We are the people Marlon Brando spoke for in the classic 1954 film *On the Waterfront* when he said, "I coulda been a contender." So many of us coulda been contenders, and shoulda been for sure.

But then, we can also make good. Can we ever! We are the seemingly tuned-out meeting participant who comes out of nowhere to provide the fresh idea that saves the day. Frequently, we are the "underachieving" child whose talent blooms with the right kind of help and finds incredible success after a checkered educational record. We *are* the contenders and the winners.

We are also imaginative and dynamic teachers, preachers, circus clowns, and stand-up comics, Navy SEALs or Army Rangers, inventors, tinkerers, and trend setters. Among us there are self-made millionaires and billionaires; Pulitzer and Nobel prize winners; Academy, Tony, Emmy, and Grammy award winners; topflight trial attorneys, brain surgeons, traders on the commodities exchange, and investment bankers. And we are often entrepreneurs. We are entrepreneurs ourselves, and the great majority of the adult patients we see for ADHD are or aspire to be entrepreneurs too. The owner and operator of an entrepreneurial support company called Strategic Coach, a man named Dan Sullivan (who also has ADHD!), estimates that at least 50 percent of his clients have ADHD as well.

Because people with ADHD don't look any different from everyone else, our condition is invisible. But if you were to climb up into our heads, you'd discover quite a different landscape. You'd find ideas firing around like kernels in a popcorn machine: ideas coming rat-a-tat fast, and on no discernable schedule. Ideas coming in spontaneous, erratic bursts. And because we can't turn this particular popcorn machine off, we are often unable to stop the idea generation at night; our minds never seem to rest.

Indeed, our minds are here and there and everywhere—all at once—which sometimes manifests as appearing to be *somewhere else,* in some dreamy state. And that means we often miss the proverbial (or literal!) boat. But then maybe we build an airplane or grab a pogo stick instead. We tune out in the middle of a job interview and don't get the job, but perhaps we see a poster hanging in the human resources waiting room that sparks a new idea that leads us to a patented invention. We offend people by forgetting names and promises, but we make good by understanding what nobody else has picked up on. We shoot ourselves in the foot, only, on the spot, to devise a painless method to remove the bullet. The great mathematician Alan Turing summed us up when he said, "Sometimes it is the people no one can imagine anything of who do the things no one can imagine." That sums us up perfectly.

Which is to say that ADHD is a far richer, more complicated, paradoxical, dangerous, but also potentially advantageous state of being than the oversimplified version most of the general public takes it to be or than even the detailed diagnostic criteria would have you believe. "ADHD" is a term that describes a way of being in the world. It is neither entirely a disorder nor entirely an asset. It is an array of traits specific to a unique kind of mind. It can become a distinct advantage or an abiding curse, depending on how a person manages it.

THE LUNATIC, THE LOVER, AND THE POET

As different as ADHD can be from person to person, there are several qualities that seem nearly universal to people with it. Distractibility, impulsivity, and hyperactivity are the classic descriptors, but they find what we think are richer and more apt counterparts in Shakespeare's musing about "the lunatic, the lover, and the poet."

Having ADHD doesn't mean you're crazy, so admittedly "lunatic" may be too strong a word. But risk taking and irrational thinking go hand in hand with ADHD behavior. *We like irrational.* We're at home in uncertainty. We're at ease where others are anxious. We're relaxed not knowing where we are or what direction we're headed in. A common lament we hear from parents of teens with ADHD makes the point: "What was he thinking? He must have lost his mind!" Likewise the spouse who asks us, "Why does he keep doing the same stupid thing over and over again? Isn't that the definition of insanity?"

Some people call this being a nonconformist, but that term misses the point. We don't *choose* not to conform. We don't even notice what the standard we're not conforming to is!

People with ADHD are lovers in the sense that they tend to have unbridled optimism. We never met a deal we didn't like, an opportunity we didn't want to pursue, a chance we didn't want to take. We get carried away. We see limitless possibilities where others see just the limits. The lover has trouble holding back, and not holding back is a major part of what it means to have ADHD.

Being a poet might best be defined with another trio of descriptors: creative, dreamy, and sometimes brooding.

"Creativity," as we use the term in connection with ADHD, designates an innate ability, desire, and irrepressible urge to plunge one's imagination regularly and deeply into life—into a project, an idea, a piece of music, a sandcastle. Indeed, people with ADHD feel an abiding need—an omnipresent itch—to create something. It's with us all the time, this unnamed appetite, whether we understand what it is or not; the act of creation offers the magnet's north pole to our south and clicks us together. It captivates us, plants us in the present, and sets us transfixed within the creative act, whatever it might happen to be.

Even awake we're dreaming, always creating, always searching for some mud pie to turn into pumpkin apple chiffon. Our imagination fuels our curiosity to find out what that noise was, or what was under the rock, or why the petri dish looks different from when we left it. If we weren't so dreamy and curious we could stay on track and never get distracted. But we do investigate the noise, the soil, the petri dish. This is why the word "deficit" in the name of our condition is such a misnomer. In fact, we do *not* suffer from a deficit of attention. Just the opposite. We've got an *overabundance* of attention, more attention than we can cope with; our constant challenge is to control it.

As for brooding, this is the special blessing and the bitter curse of ADHD. You have a vision. Maybe you've come up with a novel technology for making an unbeatable knife sharpener. Or maybe you think you have the plot to the perfect novel. Whatever your vision, you go at it like you never have before.

But then, what you've created…disappoints. It's not just disappointing, but suddenly you feel it's terrible, awful, the worst ever, and you plunge into despair. Then, just as unexpectedly, out of nowhere the vision comes back. You get reinspired. You can see it, you want it, you can't resist. You have to try again. Off you go—dreaming and creating and probably brooding again too.

Like all three characters—the lunatic, the lover, and the poet—we have a pronounced intolerance of boredom; boredom is our kryptonite. The second that we experience boredom—which you might think of as a lack of stimulation—we reflexively, instantaneously, automatically and without conscious thought seek stimulation. We don't care what it is, we just *have* to address the mental emergency—the brain pain—that boredom sets off. Like mental EMTs, we swing into action. We might pick a fight to create a bit of stimulation; we might go shopping online with manic abandon; we might rob a bank; we might snort cocaine—or we might invent the best widget the world has ever seen or come up with the solution to what's keeping our business from taking off.

PARADOXICAL TENDENCIES

We have printed the formal diagnostic definition of ADHD on page 137 so that you can see what your psychiatrist or evaluator is talking about when throwing around the diagnosis, but in less clinical terms, it helps to think of ADHD as a complex set of contradictory or paradoxical tendencies: a lack of focus combined with an ability to superfocus; a lack of direction combined with highly directed entrepreneurialism; a tendency to procrastinate combined with a knack for getting a week's worth of work done in two hours; impulsive, wrongheaded decision making combined with inventive, out-of-the-blue problem solving; interpersonal cluelessness combined with uncanny intuition and empathy; the list goes on.

Here, more formally, are the telltale signs of ADHD that might send you looking for clinical confirmation:

Unexplained underachievement. The person is simply not doing as well as innate talent and brainpower warrant. There's no obvious explanation, like poor eyesight, serious physical illness, or cognitive impairment due to head injury, say.

A wandering mind. You'll get frequent comments from teachers, or, in an adult, supervisors or spouse, that the individual's mind wanders, that he or she has trouble focusing and staying on task, that performance is inconsistent, good days and bad days, good moments and terrible ones, all of which usually lead the teacher, supervisor, or spouse to conclude that the person in question needs more discipline, needs to try harder, needs to learn to *pay attention.* No kidding! But such is the ignorance that still surrounds ADHD that people continue to cite lack of effort as the cause of the disorganization and poor attention. The biological fact is that, in the absence of stimulation, they *can't*. Not won't. *Can't*.

Trouble organizing and planning. In the clinical jargon, this is called trouble with "executive function." The child, say, has trouble getting dressed in the morning. You can ask your daughter to go upstairs and get dressed only to find her fifteen minutes later still in her nightclothes, lying on her bed engrossed in a conversation with her doll. Or you can ask your husband to take out the trash and in the time it takes him to walk over to the trash container, he forgets what he's supposed to be doing and slowly ambles *right past it*. You go ballistic, believing your husband is being blatantly provocative, passive-aggressive, oppositional, or colossally self-centered, all adjectives you've applied to him hundreds of times in the past. Before you get divorced, it would be marriage-saving if someone could explain to you both that walking past the trash, like hundreds of other acts of seemingly selfish disregard for others, stems not from selfishness or another character defect but from a neurological condition that renders attention inconsistent and immediate memory so porous that a task can be forgotten in a heartbeat. What compounds these problems, and makes some people doubt the validity of the diagnosis, is that these same people can hyperfocus, deliver a brilliant presentation on time, and be super-reliable *when they are stimulated.* But, as we've said, boredom is kryptonite; the ADHD mind recoils from boredom, disappearing into a fervent search for stimulation while the trash can sits forlornly unemptied.

High degree of creativity and imagination. People with ADHD—at any age—often possess intellectual effervescence. Unfortunately, this natural sparkle can be snuffed out by years of criticism, reprimands, redirection, lack of appreciation, and repeated disappointments, frustrations, and outright failures.

Trouble with time management, and a tendency to procrastinate. This is another element of executive function, and quite an interesting one. Those of us who have ADHD experience time differently from other people. This is *really* hard for most people to believe, which is why people are typically unsympathetic to our problem and ascribe it to lack of effort, a bad attitude, or pure obstinacy. But the fact is that we lack an internal sense of the arc of time; we're unaware of the unstoppable flow of seconds into minutes into hours, days, and so forth. Defying the laws of physics, we change the nature of time in our minds. In our world, we have little awareness of the seconds ticking by; few internal alerts, alarms, or cues; no judicious allocation of chunks of time for this, then that, and then the next thing. We short-circuit all such complexity by slicing time down to its barest bones. In our world, we recognize only two times: "now" and "not now." We hear "We have to leave in a half hour" as "We don't have to leave now." "The paper is due in five days" becomes "It's not due now," and the five days might as well be five months. We hear "I'll have to go to bed sometime" when someone has actually said "It's time for bed now." Our truncated sense of time leads to all manner of fights, failures, job losses, disappointed friends, and failed romances, but at the same time to an uncanny ability to work brilliantly under extreme pressure, as well as to be wonderfully, infuriatingly oblivious to the time pressures that stress most people to the max.

Strong will, stubbornness, refusal of help. It can seem stunningly stupid, but many people with ADHD, especially men, state outright, "I'd rather fail doing it my way than succeed with help."

Generosity. As painful as the distortions we carry around can be, we also carry around a pocketful of miracles, a positive energy that comes and goes. But when it comes, we are the most generous people you'll ever find, the most optimistic, the most enthusiastic. Yes, ironically, although we tend to reject help from others (see above!), we are the ones who offer the shirt off our back to the person who needs it, whether we know them or not. It's why so many of us excel in sales. We can be charismatic, infectiously funny, persuasive, and just what you need if you're feeling low.

Restlessness, especially in boys and men. *Woolgathering,* especially in girls and women. Because they tend not to be hyperactive or disruptive, females of all ages remain the most undiagnosed group. You have to be a savvy parent, teacher, spouse, supervisor, or doctor to pick up inattentive, non-hyperactive ADHD in a girl or woman.

Unique and active sense of humor. Quirky, offbeat, but usually rather sophisticated too. Many stand-up comics and comedy writers have ADHD, perhaps in part because of our fundamentally different ways of seeing the world. We live outside the proverbial box. In fact, one of us probably invented the psychological test that the phrase "thinking outside the box" comes from.

Trouble sharing and playing with others early on, but at the same time, a desire to make friends. As life progresses, social problems can develop, due to trouble reading the social scene and inability to control the impulse to interrupt or butt in. In adulthood, this translates to seeming gruff, awkward, rude, self-centered, unfiltered, or aloof; but it is really just the undiagnosed and untreated ADHD that is causing the problems. This is why we call ADHD such a "good news" diagnosis: Once you know you have it, and you find the right help, life can only get better, often *much* better.

Exquisite sensitivity to criticism or rejection. William Dodson, one of the smartest clinicians ever to write about ADHD, made famous the term "rejection-sensitive dysphoria," or RSD, which describes a tendency on the part of people who have ADHD to overreact precipitously and disastrously to even the slightest perceived put-down, dis, or vaguely negative remark. They can spiral down to the depths in the blink of an eye and become inconsolable. On the other hand (there's *always* an *other* hand in this syndrome so characterized by pairs of opposite symptoms), we've coined another term to describe the opposite of RSD. It is "recognition-sensitive euphoria," or RSE, which refers to our enhanced ability to make constructive use of praise, affirmation, and encouragement. As much as we can get down in the dumps over a minute criticism, we can fly high and put to great use even small bits of encouragement or recognition.

Impulsiveness and impatience. We make quick decisions and have trouble delaying gratification. We flunk the marshmallow test.[*1] We tend to operate on a "fire, aim, ready" basis instead of "ready, aim, fire." But remember, the flip side of impulsivity is creativity. Creativity is impulsivity gone right. You do not *plan* to have a creative idea, a eureka moment, a sudden revelation. These all come without bidding or warning. They come to us *impulsively.*

An itch to change the conditions of life. As you get older, this tends to manifest as a general dissatisfaction with ordinary life leading to a need to improve upon it, augment it, supercharge it, ratchet it up several notches. This "itch" can lead to major achievements and creations, or it can lead to addictions of all kinds as well as a host of other dangerous behaviors.

Often it leads to both.

High energy (hence the use of "hyperactivity" in the disorder name), coupled with a tendency toward lassitude, often mistaken for laziness.

Uncannily accurate intuition, coupled with a tendency to overlook the obvious and ignore major data.

Transparency, to the point of being honest to a fault. The person who is incapable of "kissing up," intolerant of hypocrisy, often tactless, politically incorrect, and heedless of repercussions and consequences...is often dealing with ADHD. On the other hand, especially in children, this translates into a tendency to lie impulsively when put on the spot. This is not a character defect or a lack of conscience, which we see in a sociopath, but rather a reflexive attempt to change reality, as in wishing it were so.

Susceptibility to addictions and compulsive behaviors of all kinds. From drugs and alcohol, to gambling, shopping, spending, sex, food, exercise, and screens, we who have ADHD are five to ten times more likely than the person who does not have ADHD to develop a problem in this domain. This stems from the "itch" mentioned earlier and the need to juice up reality. The upside of this symptom is that if you find the right creative outlet—start a business, write a book, build a house, plant a garden—you can scratch the itch that way, rather than develop a bad habit or an outright addiction.

Having a metaphorical lightning rod and weather vane. For whatever reason, people with ADHD often are lightning rods for whatever can go wrong: being the one kid caught with weed when twenty others had it; the adult or kid who gets scapegoated, blamed, and disciplined more than anyone else; the one who disrupts the family event, or business meeting, or class discussion without meaning to. But at the same time, the lightning rod quality can lead the person with ADHD to receive ideas, energies, premonitions, and images from who knows where that lead to amazing success. Similarly, the internal, inborn weather vane leads the person with ADHD to be the first to sense a shift in mood or energy in the group, the class, the family, the organization, the town, the country. Before others catch on, the person with ADHD is telling others to watch out, there's an ill wind brewing; or to get ready, a big opportunity is just around the corner. Like the lightning rod, the weather vane effect can't be explained on any scientific basis we know of, but we see it in our patients, of all ages, all the time.

Tendency to externalize or blame others while not seeing your role in the problem. This is coupled with a general inability to observe oneself accurately, which naturally leads to more externalizing, since you truly do not see the role you play in the problem.

Distorted negative self-image. Due to the inability to observe oneself accurately, coupled with the heightened sensitivity to perceived criticism and a record of underachievement, people with ADHD usually have a self-image that is far more negative than is warranted. One of our patients calls the condition "attention deficit distorter" because of how it distorts so many perceptions of reality. While on the one hand, creativity depends upon the ability to imagine a different reality, to "distort" the ordinary into something better, on the other hand, this "distorter" can create one of the most painful aspects of ADHD, which is very low self-regard. We look at ourselves as if in a house of mirrors, not seeing ourselves as others do, seeing only what we regard as failures and shortcomings, all but blind to the upside, which is typically considerable. We suffer shame as we misread ourselves and misread others' responses to us. We hold back on opportunities and relationships out of that shame, as well as fear and misunderstanding.

BIOLOGICAL OR CULTURALLY INDUCED ADHD?

Scientific estimates suggest that between 5 and 10 percent of people are born with some combination of the characteristics we have just listed. This number represents those of us born with ADHD. As such, it is actually recognized as one of the most heritable conditions in the behavioral sciences. "Heritable" means you inherit a collection of genes that increase the likelihood that you will develop a condition during your lifetime. Though it might be helpful to be able to identify just which genes are involved in ADHD, the reality is that there is no one or two genes for ADHD but an array, which makes sense, given that ADHD is a coat of so many colors.

If one parent has ADHD, the risk is one in three that a given child will have ADHD. If both parents have ADHD, the risk is two in three for a given child. However, those are just averages. In Dr. Hallowell's family, for example, he has ADHD, his wife does not, but all three of their children have it.

In addition to genetics, we've also known for a long time that certain environmental stressors can cause ADHD, most notably head injuries or lack of oxygen at birth, early infections, or any other brain insult. (A "brain insult," by the way, is not someone telling you that you have an ugly brain, but your brain's function being in some way interfered with such as by fever, toxins like lead or mercury, or trauma.)

We've also known that a mother's being obese or drinking alcohol, using drugs, or smoking cigarettes during pregnancy can raise the risk of the baby's developing ADHD. Still unproven, but being studied vis-à-vis neurological functioning, is another risk factor we might add to the list: magnetic field non-ionizing radiation (MFR), which comes in two forms, low frequency and high frequency. Low frequency MFR comes from, among other sources, power lines and kitchen appliances. High frequency MFR, the newer one, comes from wireless networks and cellphones. Stay tuned…

—

Beyond the sources of biologically based ADHD, there are a lot of people who act as if they have ADHD but on close inspection turn out not to have the diagnosable condition. These are the people who have ADHD-like symptoms caused by the conditions of modern life. Their "ADHD" is a response to the massive increase in stimuli that now bombard our brains and our world.

The massive behavioral conditioning we've all been undergoing since the advent of ubiquitous electronic communications technology has changed us radically. But this dramatic, if not epochal, change is underappreciated. It's underappreciated because we're living in it as it happens, like frogs in cold water that slowly gets heated up without the frogs trying to jump out, until they're boiled. Our world has been getting heated up big-time. And while we *could* jump out, it's pretty difficult to do so and still function in the modern world. Modern life has trained our brains to go faster and faster, to do more and more, to receive and transmit 24/7, and to require constant stimulation—be it from movies, TV, conversation, even news, as well as the minute-to-minute living of our lives. Most of us can go no more than a few seconds without looking for a screen.

Modern life compels these changes by forcing our brains to process exponentially more data points than ever before in human history, dramatically more than we did prior to the era of the Internet, smartphones, and social media. The hardwiring of our brains has not changed—as far as we know, although some experts do suspect that our hardwiring is changing—but in our efforts to adapt to the speeding up of life and the projectile spewing of data splattering onto our brains all the time, we've had to develop new, often rather antisocial habits in order to cope. These habits have come together to create something we now call VAST: the *variable attention stimulus trait.*[*2]

Whether you have true ADHD or its environmentally induced cousin, VAST, it's important to detoxify the label and focus on the inherent positives. To be clear, we don't want you to deny there is a downside to what you are going through, but we want you also to identify the upside.

In the descriptors we offer for VAST below, you will see there is no requirement for impairment, because we are not designating this as a disorder, but as a trait. You will note there is also mention of many strengths. And unlike a formal ADHD diagnosis, for which six out of nine criteria on the axis of inattention or the axis of hyperactivity and impulsivity need to be present (see appendix A for a full listing of these symptoms), there is no set number of descriptors to qualify for the diagnosis, or what we prefer to call the "description" or "self-portrait."

In fact, the diagnostic criteria for ADHD found in DSM-5, the official diagnostic manual, have inadvertently created a lot of confusion. People often ask, "Do I have ADD or ADHD?" Technically, there is no longer any such thing as ADD. You can only have ADHD. But there are qualifiers. If you have at least six out of nine symptoms on the axis of inattention, but not on the axis of hyperactivity and impulsivity, then you have *ADHD, predominantly inattentive.* This is what used to be called ADD. If you have six out of nine symptoms on both axes, then you have *ADHD, combined* type. And if you are one of the extremely rare people who has symptoms only on the axis of hyperactivity and impulsivity, then you have *ADHD, predominantly hyperactive-impulsive.*

For the variable attention stimulus trait, we do not call what we offer below "diagnostic criteria" at all. Instead, if you see yourself in the following list of descriptors enough that they describe you and set you apart from others, well, then, VAST fits you, and what we have to say about how to live best with this trait may be useful to you.

Last, in the chart we have created in the pages that follow, you'll quickly see that there is an opposite word to each descriptor. That's because, like ADHD, VAST is a condition of paradoxical pairs, ups and downs, lefts and rights. That's why living with it can be such a mishmash, so confusing, but also so exciting and at times groundbreaking. (You'll also note that there is a lot of overlap among the twenty descriptors of ADHD.)

USEFUL	PROBLEMATIC
Passionate; zealous; idealistic; will sacrifice everything for a cause or a friend	Can become rigid in the service of a cause; can become fanatical, strident, irrational; Captain Ahab syndrome
Meticulous at times, especially on projects that matter a great deal	Usually disorganized, even chaotically so; chaos can rule to such an extent that school, job, marriage hang in balance
Can get a lot done in a short amount of time	Fundamentally different sense of time; there is only NOW and NOT NOW in this world, so procrastination rules, and things rarely get done on time
An appreciation of the offbeat, unusual, unconventional	An inability or refusal to conform or get in line when doing so is obviously in his or her best interest
Dreamer par excellence; visionary; lives on wings of imagination, flights of fancy	Sometimes so bored by reality that he or she ignores it and gets into trouble for having done so
Honest to a fault; will say what others don't dare to say; outspoken; blunt	Can hurt feelings and damage self; can unwittingly be cruel, which is last thing he or she wants to be
Intense desire to be free and independent, own boss; master of own fate	Trouble working on teams; trouble taking orders; trouble with intimacy in private life
Naturally creative; ideas pop all the time like in a popcorn machine	Trouble organizing all the ideas and doing something productive with them

Naturally curious; always wanting to know who, what, where, why, and how; never satisfied until he or she gets the answer	Easily distracted by novelty or any puzzle, conundrum, unsolved problem, or beguiling opportunity, however irrelevant it may be
Enormously energetic; seemingly indefatigable	Impulsive; can't sit still or linger over a conversation or ponder an idea with a colleague or a relative
Mind like a steel trap; can remember details from years ago	Forgets what he or she went into the next room to get; forgets where he or she put car keys; forgets wallet, glasses, umbrella; leaves groceries on roof of car and drives off
Full of ideas	So many ideas they choke the growth of any single one
Decisive; can make an important, complex decision in a split second	Impatient; hates to wrestle with ambiguity; shoots from the hip
Initial surge of excitement over new plan, deal, idea, project, relationship	Excitement peters out in the middle phase; trouble sustaining interest
Takes responsibility; gets done what needs to get done	Trouble delegating, trusting that others can do it as well as he or she can
Tenacious; never gives up; will literally collapse before quitting	Stubborn; would rather fail doing it his or her way than succeed taking advice from someone else; can spend a lifetime trying to get good at what he or she's bad at
Can act on the spur of the moment	Procrastination can be a huge problem
Original; sees solutions others do not; comes up with novel ideas	Can seem whacky, eccentric, even crazy; can put people off by being too offbeat and arrogant
Confident; self-assured	Insecure; despite confident exterior feels success was all done by smoke and mirrors
Extremely hardworking	Driven; compulsive; can't let up; maniacal
Lightning-quick mind	Trouble shutting mind down; risk of developing addictions to quiet mind down
Risk taker; focuses and performs best in situations of crisis and danger	Needs danger in order to feel engaged with life and truly alive
Sees the big picture before anyone else	Trouble with implementation and sweating the details
Generous; bighearted; willing to give with no expectation of return	Can give away the store
Funny; the life of the party; can connect with everyone	Secretly lonely; feels no one really knows him
Innovator	Can't/won't follow instructions

Pays close attention when interested	Easily distracted; mind wanders when not interested; frequently on electronic devices and difficult to engage
Supremely talented in several domains	Seriously limited in several domains
A life enthusiast; wants to try everything; can't ever get enough	Overcommitted; about to snap
Strong leader; charismatic	Hates the position of leader; worries he or she will let everyone down; unaware of his or her own charisma
Thrives in highly stimulating situations	Finds contentment too bland and so can disrupt ordinary happiness in order to create high stimulation
Loves debate, conflict, sparring	Intimacy can be difficult unless partner likes these as well

*1 In 1972, the Stanford psychologist Walter Mischel devised an experiment using marshmallows to test a child's ability to delay gratification.

*2 Carrie Feibel, health editor at KQED in San Francisco, suggested the phrase and acronym to us. We liked it so much that we adopted it, with her permission.

CHAPTER 2

Understanding the Demon of the Mind

Imagine a man named Hank. Hank is a natural-born salesman, good with people, a good judge of character.

But Hank is also tortured, and that's not too strong a word for the mental miseries he endures. He spends chunks of time—fifteen minutes here, an hour there, sometimes an entire Saturday morning and even longer—*brooding*. Troubling, jagged thoughts, images, ideas, and feelings pop up unimpeded in his mind like rocks in a river's current as he desperately tries to steady his mental raft. They keep on coming, smashing against his mind over and over while he bravely tries to survive another trip down the relentlessly moving rapids within.

Fixed in place by the torrent of his negative thoughts, Hank sits in the easy chair in his living room, feet on the floor, fingers digging into the arms of his chair, staring out the window at a sunny afternoon. Of course he does see what's actually outside—an elm tree in the foreground, the street beyond—but he can't really take in the view. All he sees is danger and more metaphorical rocks to get past.

This horrible ruminative process is as much a routine part of Hank's life as brushing his teeth or commuting to work. Only it lasts longer and it produces only pain, no gain.

Now forty years old, Hank is underachieving at work, not because he lacks talent—he has talent coming out his ears, as his boss said—but because he "just can't get his act together," to quote his exasperated wife.

Hank is more exasperated than anyone, which only fuels his incessant self-recrimination. He's tried antidepressants, which did nothing but reduce his libido, diminishing one of the few pleasures in his life. He's tried psychotherapy, which ironically caused him guilt because he felt he was frustrating the psychologist and making the psychologist feel incompetent. "It's not your fault, doc," he said in their final meeting, the one in which Hank declared himself incurable. "I'm just wired differently. I've got the devil of a dark side. I might as well get used to it."

Like many people, Hank experiences excessive worry. But because he also has ADHD, his worry has been magnified. Ironically for a condition commonly associated with lack of focus, many people with ADHD—or with the VAST characteristics—focus on their worry so much that it wears a rut in their thinking. And like a rut in the road, it can be hard to avoid. Fortunately, we now know how these ruts get made and how to steer the mind out of them.

NEW FINDINGS, NEW HELP

Enter one of our world's greatest triumphs of the past thirty years: advances in brain science. After millennia of moral (*It's all a matter of willpower; suck it up*); religious (*Give your suffering up to God* or *"Whate'er He gives, He gives the best"*); or philosophical (*Control what you can, accept what you can't*) explanations and remedies for mental anguish, we now live in an era when we can assess the actual substrate in which the action occurs, namely, your brain and its attendant nervous system.

We can now measure the many molecules in the brain; the electrical activity; the flow of blood; the differential consumption of glucose (energy) and oxygen; and the actual size of various regions of the brain and correlate the size with the function of that area. We're starting to understand the genetics behind brain function, as well as the epigenetics, the varying impact of environment upon the expression of genes.

For example, it is because of epigenetics that you may have been born with genes that predispose you to depression, but because of loving parents and a nurturing school system, those genes never get expressed. You go through life never suffering from depression, even though you carry the genes that might have led you there. On the other hand, if you had unloving parents, if you never received nurturing and positive connections, or, worse, if you suffered trauma and abuse, then if you also inherited the genes that predispose you to depression or other pathology, those genes are far more likely to get expressed. Regardless of the trait, condition, disorder, or disease, nature versus nurture *always* comes down to *both.* Good nurture can dramatically reduce the influence of bad nature, bad genes; unfortunately, the reverse is also true: bad nurture, like cold or distant parents, ongoing conflict, or outright trauma while growing up, can suppress good nature, good genes.

The science of epigenetics has helped prove the brain's wondrous ability to change over the course of your lifetime. Called *neuroplasticity,* this is one of the major discoveries in neuroscience in the past generation. People used to believe that the brain was more or less set by a certain age—let's say thirty— and after that the die was cast, the brain was set.

This fixed-brain notion begat a host of homespun clichés and conventional wisdom to the effect that you simply cannot teach an old dog, or even a middle-aged dog, new tricks; that from age thirty the leopard does not change its spots, that you are who you are and you better get used to it because no amount of therapy, life experience, or other magic can make a significant dent in the architecture of your brain or your personality, except by changing it for the worse, through disease, stroke, cancer, poisons, alcohol, drugs, or dementia.

Wrong. As with much homespun wisdom regarding the mind, we now know different. Thanks to the work of many neuroscientists, we know that what you do, who you love, where you live, what you eat, how much you move, what kind of stress you experience, if you have a pet, whether you laugh a lot—all those and a zillion more bits of experience constantly change who you are in subtle ways. Your brain responds to all these cues in turn.

Most people do not realize what fantastically great news this is. We *can* change who we are and where we're headed. It's not easy, but it can be done, and done at any age. You're never too old to find a new life, a new love, a better day. Our brains present us with the opportunity day in and day out. We just have to unwrap the gift.

The science of the last thirty years also explains, at least in part, the tension and the contradictions that lie at the core of ADHD and VAST. It explains what's going on in our brains that leads to creativity, entrepreneurialism, and dynamism, but also, at the same time, irrational brooding, worrying, ruminating, and falling prey to self-destructive addictions and compulsions. If Hank had known about all this, he might have been able to circumvent his tortured thoughts. He also could have started to use his talents—empathy, emotional intelligence, and creativity—to excel in his chosen profession.

BRAIN BASICS

In chapter 1 we stressed that ADHD is a syndrome of contradictions and paradoxes. Each negative has a matched positive and vice versa. You can focus, but then not focus, or you're forced into hyperfocus when you don't want to be. We emphasized the inconsistency created by the brain's dueling banjos, so to speak, and how ADHD is never all good or all bad. Now we can explain why this is so.

Central to both the gift of creativity and the curse of brooding lie two mindsets we like to call the Angel and the Demon. These are not at all religious references. We think of them more like the benevolent spirit that whispers encouragement from one shoulder and the imp on the other who gives terrible advice. The Angel bestows the gifts, and the Demon casts the curse. With practical tools, you can learn to activate the Angel while shutting down the Demon—often without medication.

To unpack all this, let's begin with some nuts-and-bolts explanations that apply to everyone, VAST, ADHD, or "neurotypical," as we say in psychiatry.

When you are engaged in a task of any kind, from frying an egg to writing an email to digging a hole, various clumps of neurons, together called a *connectome,* "light up" in your brain. We can see this through the exciting new science of fMRI, or functional magnetic resonance imaging. It's like a live, moving X-ray, and it's as close as we now can get to watching thought in motion.

The connectome that lights up when you're engaged in a task is called the *task-positive network,* or TPN. Aptly named, the TPN gets you down to work. You're deliberately doing something and you are intent on it, unaware of much beyond the bounds of what you're doing. In this state, you don't consciously know whether you're happy or not, which is just as good as being happy, if not better, because you're not wasting any energy in self-assessment. You may become frustrated with what you're doing and have moments of anger or dismay, but if you stay in the task, in the TPN, those moments will pass, and the TPN, buoyant connectome that it is, will carry you along. When you're thinking with the TPN, you're in the Angel mindset. But you can also get trapped in the TPN, doing a task from which you cannot disengage. This is the hyperfocused state that people with ADHD can fall into. Far from being helpful, it can keep you stuck in one task, unable to shut down the screen, turn off the TV, or move from one paragraph to the next. This is the often unrecognized downside of focus.

Incidentally, the reason that so many people are starting to look and act distracted, as if they all have ADHD or VAST, is that fewer and fewer people are spending time in the task-positive network. They are not spending enough time focusing on a single task, certainly not long enough to dig a deep enough hole or write an email longer than a sentence or two or do more than look at an egg, let alone fry one. Unfortunately, the TPN is akin to a muscle that atrophies when not used. So as we mentally flit around, the TPN weakens and our attention span shortens.

When you allow your mind to wander from a task, or when you finish the task, or if you pause too long in anger or dismay while doing the task, the TPN in your brain defaults to a different connectome. Not surprisingly—given that we default to this state—this other connectome is called the *default mode network* (DMN). The DMN allows for expansive, imaginative, and creative thinking. The back half of the DMN—called the *posterior cingulate*—facilitates your autobiographic memory, your personal history. This allows you to think back, draw upon, and pick apart the past. The front part, the *medial prefrontal cortex,* is the opposite. It enables you to look forward and to think about, imagine, and plan for the future.

It is in the DMN mode that you can daydream (and miss your exit on the highway) or make interesting connections between concepts (helpful when appreciating riddles or jokes or solving crossword puzzles, or coming up with the Next Big Thing). It was surely in the DMN that the wheel was discovered!

The DMN and TPN are the yin and yang of your brain. Both help us and hold us back in certain ways. One isn't better than the other. But as helpful as the DMN can be (angelic in its own right), it is also a Demon (as its initialism suggests!) for the ADHD or VAST brain because of our capacity for intractable rumination while captive in it.

THE GLITCHY SWITCH

For neurotypical people, toggling over to the DMN periodically allows you to get some intellectual rest and relaxation—daydreaming time, for instance, which isn't necessarily bad. But highly imaginative, creative people—like those of us who have ADHD or VAST—often get *stuck* in the DMN, leading to horribly negative, gloomy, and self-critical thoughts like the ones we saw in Hank's experience earlier.

While we are all wired to feel fear and imagine disaster far more than to feel comfortable and secure (along with our five senses, the imagination is our chief evolutionary danger detector), people who have ADHD or VAST are also particularly prone to head toward gloom and doom in their minds because they have stored up in their memory banks a lifetime of moments of failure, disappointment, shame, frustration, defeat, and embarrassment. Given a moment to reflect on what's likely to happen next, life has taught people with ADHD to imagine and expect the worst. Too many facts are readily available to support the thesis that, well, life sucks.

The cutting-edge work of a neuroscientist and professor at MIT named John Gabrieli points up another reason that people with ADHD or the variable attention stimulus trait are more prone to negativity.

"I think of the Default Mode Network as our internal self-system," says

Gabrieli. "It's a bit of a chatterbox." Some chatter is good, some is destructive.

To paraphrase Gabrieli, the problem when ADHD enters in is twofold. The first is what's called the *anticorrelation property* of the two networks. Imagine a seesaw. In a neurotypical brain, when the TPN is turned on and you're on task, the DMN is turned off. But in the ADHD brain, the fMRI shows that when the TPN is turned on, *the DMN is turned on as well,* trying to muscle its way in and pull you into its grasp, thereby distracting you. *In ADHD, therefore, the DMN competes with the TPN, which in most people it does not do.*

Adding another important spin, Gabrieli says that within the DMN itself, between the front and back regions, the opposite occurs: "Typically, people have synchrony in their default mode network. They go up and down together. Not so in the ADHD brain. They are off-kilter, out of sync." That's what's meant by anticorrelation. Instead of working in unison, they work against each other.

If that's not complicated enough, Gabrieli explains an even more important issue undermining the ADHD brain. It's how these networks interact, both internally and with each other.

Adjusting his glasses, he makes his strongest point:

"If there is one takeaway in distilling down the complexity of the DMN and the TPN, it boils down to the fact that the toggle switches between them are off in those with ADHD."

In other words, in most people the DMN does not slip so easily into the TPN; the gears mesh well and are not glitchy. But in people who have ADHD, the gears get stripped, so to speak, and so you're left with this dangerous/wonderful curse/gift. This is truly a malfunction of the imagination, and it explains the confluence of the creative and depressive we so often see within the same person, even within the same hour.

The creative side gains expression and something beautiful takes shape. But then the depressive side carps, "That's ugly. You've failed again." The creative side sinks under the weight until its natural resilience and buoyancy— or the glitchy switch—brings it back with a bang.

The blessing and the curse vie for top billing, for attention. When the DMN brings lovely images, it is our golden tool. But when it jumps track into the TPN and hijacks consciousness, then the DMN becomes the Demon, the seat of misery, the disease of the imagination. Trapped in the past or future in the DMN, you're likely to abandon projects you once started with enthusiasm, make careless mistakes, or, worse, fall into a state of misery and despair, for no good reason whatsoever.

All creative people can recognize only too well the phenomenon of being on a roll—creating—only to have a negative voice trying to interrupt the process. That's the faulty "toggle switch" allowing the DMN to intrude on the TPN. Being trapped in it is painful; the term "tortured artist" fits. Indeed, many of our greatest scientists, inventors, performers, and writers have struggled with glitchy connections, vacillating between creating great works and languishing in despair, often seeking relief in drugs, alcohol, or self-destructive compulsive activity.

ADHD AND ADDICTION

When the DMN rules, it demands *more*. This hunger can be satisfied through artistic achievement or through entrepreneurial wheeling and dealing or, maybe best of all, through love. But if and when these efforts don't pay off— the novel you're writing doesn't resonate with readers, the deal falls through, the relationship ends—you have to start the search again for how you will bring ordinary life sufficiently alive to satisfy the hunger of your imagination.

While this hunger can lead to magnificent achievements of many kinds, in the extreme, *this exact same hunger drives addiction.* That's why addictions of all kinds are five to ten times more common in people who have ADHD than in the general population. We live with an itch at our core that can only be scratched in certain ways. Creative achievement is perhaps the most adaptive, worthwhile, and sustainable, while addictions—of all kinds—are the most maladaptive and destructive.

All of this goes a long way toward explaining the truism so often observed that creative talent goes hand in hand with addiction, depression, bipolar disorder, ADHD, and all manner of mental disturbance. It's largely a function of the overlap of the Angel and the Demon, the glitchy connections that appear in this part of the brain in highly creative people, certainly in people who've been studied with classically defined ADHD. Though the connection has not been formally researched, we see people with the variable attention stimulus trait (VAST) in our practices who are increasingly struggling with addictions too.

THE GLITCHY SWITCH IN ACTION

Now that you know a little bit about glitchy connections and faulty toggle switches in the ADHD brain, you can start to recognize when you or a loved one is stuck, and what part of the brain is taking hold. This is of enormous *practical* value, not just academic interest, which we will get into later.

But first, an illustration. John Ratey's uncle Ron. While he is, sadly, no longer with us, the stories surrounding his ADHD are legendary within the family and live on in affectionate retelling at holiday gatherings. A beloved elementary school teacher, Ron raised four kids with his wife, Gretchen, whom he adored.

One year, in celebration of the arrival of spring after a cold winter, Ron and Gretchen set out to the hardware store to get flowers and plants for the front yard, along with a few other supplies for the house. Pulling in to the parking lot, they got out of the car and decided to divide and conquer, with Ron getting the plants and Gretchen setting off to the plumbing department. With enthusiastic zeal, Uncle Ron made a beeline for the gardening section. He jumped deep into his DMN, envisioning how each type of flower and foliage would look in the front yard, making mental notes on where his shovel and planting tools were in the garage, and daydreaming about how beautiful the yard would look after it was all finished.

Once home, digging in the dirt, Ron moved squarely into his task mode to a fault, methodically plotting out the perfect distance between the plants, creating exacting, uniform holes, taking care to watch the roots as he pulled the plants from the plastic containers.

This continued until his teenaged daughter, Renee, came out the front door.

"Dad, where's Mom?" she asked.

It took a minute to sink in. Uncle Ron suddenly realized that he had left Gretchen at the store. When he left the parking lot, he was so focused in the front part of his DMN, planning for the future, envisioning his garden, that he didn't connect to the back part of his DMN, the history that revealed he had a wife he adored, and the memory that they had driven to the store together.

If you think he panicked, apologizing profusely, thinking about the love of his life stranded and alone, you would be wrong. Uncle Ron was now so deep in his TPN, focusing on the singular task of taking his plantings to the finish line, he continued to carefully smooth the dirt around a peony with one hand while tossing his keys to Renee with the other, instructing her to take the car to get her mother.

"But, Dad," said Renee, "I just have my learner's permit. I can't drive alone."

Uncle Ron was very involved with and loved his kids. He frequently rode shotgun with Renee as she learned to drive on side roads and in parking lots. At this point in our story, he had actually arranged for her to have a driving test the following week, so he clearly knew she only had a learner's permit. But his brain was so rigidly focused on his task of planting his flowers that it was not easily connecting to those historical facts in his DMN.

Leaving Gretchen stranded wasn't an isolated incident.

Gretchen was a substitute teacher, and when she got an assignment at a nearby school, Ron often dropped her off before continuing on to his own job. More than once, he walked through the front door at the end of the day, only to be met with sickening silence and the realization he had forgotten to pick up his wife where he'd left her that morning.

It was not until years later, when their son was being tested for ADHD, that Ron discovered his own. Explaining that ADHD tends to run in families, the psychiatrist inquired if Ron wanted to take a test as well. As you might expect, he was off the charts with his diagnosis.

While you might have smiled appreciatively at Uncle Ron's story, the consequences of having faulty, glitchy connections in your brain can sometimes be much more devastating and exhausting than just your spouse's inconvenience. It can seriously affect schoolwork, your job, your relationships, and your overall feeling of well-being. Those of us with ADHD or VAST battle constant frustration from being two steps behind (not to mention the ire of those we are behind) because we're trapped in one area of the brain or another.

Another extremely common problem when caught in the DMN is what we call "pirouette syndrome," a circling back to make *sure* you've done something you've already done. Some people pirouette to be sure they've locked the front door, or didn't leave eggs boiling on the stove; others circle back to find something they are sure they've forgotten: sunglasses, a wallet. When you aren't paying attention in your TPN, it takes a lot of energy to check and double-check to make sure you didn't pull a royal screw-up. Chances are you did lock the door, took the eggs off the stove, and had your sunglasses on top of your head, but because you weren't focused in the moment, niggling doubt keeps you panicked until you can go back and check.

Still another curse of the Demon is catastrophic thinking. We refer to this as Chicken Little syndrome, as it's easy to believe the sky is falling. A young attorney confessed she has a tough time starting new cases as she immediately jumps to the future part of her DMN and stays there, endlessly envisioning and obsessing about what can go wrong with her argument, the five thousand ways her client might misbehave, the ten thousand ways she might blow it with the jury. As she knows only too well, while it is always good to develop options in case things go wrong, if you stay there too long, you can't focus on the task at hand and work effectively toward preventing those mistakes.

Of course, catastrophic thinking is a form of rumination. Your boss throws off a comment that you perceive as a slight. The rear part of the DMN spins into overdrive, looking back at what she said, taking it apart, wondering what you did to deserve that. Was it really a pointed dig? Then you beat yourself up, thinking back, ruminating on what you might have said or done to provoke the comment. You take apart every imperfect thing you said or did at work, reliving the embarrassment. There's more than enough angst to go around.

Then there's the front part of the DMN, where you ruminate on plans and make lists. You go over and over and over what you will say to your boss to straighten things out, or how you will chastise her and quit, stressing about her reaction, your cowardice, and the fallout. You're convinced you're going to screw it up, as this is the part of the brain that projects humiliating occurrences happening again.

THE CLEVER ART OF OUTSMARTING THE DEMON

There's a famous saying among neuroscientists: Neurons that fire together, wire together. To be sure, when you're ruminating, you're repeatedly doing something that fosters a *negative* connection over time. But this neurological understanding shines a light on the solution as well: If neurons that fire together, wire together (making increasingly permanent connections), you need to fire them in another direction. The trick is to take advantage of the fact that the DMN can jump tracks. Because if it can run to darkness, well, then, we can make it jump tracks and run to the light. Two can play at this game!

In other words: *Spend more time in the TPN focusing on a single task.* We know what you might be thinking: *The whole point is that I* can't *focus on a single task!* But you can—you are already a master of distraction, so now distract *yourself*. Productivity isn't the point here. Moving the toggle switch is.

As a practical matter, this means that the minute you start to ruminate and slip into brooding negativity, look elsewhere. Do anything. Walk around. Yell. Dance a jig. Dice celery. Play the piano. Feed your dog. Sing "Row, Row, Row Your Boat" while standing on one leg. Tie your shoes. Whistle "Dixie." Blow your nose. Jump rope. Bark like a dog, howl like a wolf, call a radio show and vent like a maniac. Do a crossword. Work your brain. Read a book. Hell, why not *write* a book? Sure, dig a hole or fry a few eggs. Or try an exercise that zeroes in on your breathing. Pick a pattern to focus on, for example, 6-3-8-3. Inhale for six beats, hold for three, exhale for eight beats, hold for three; repeat. After a few cycles, you will move out of the DMN.

The point is: *Focus on anything external to yourself. Activating the TPN will shut down the DMN.* It's difficult to do because the DMN is seductive and the negative messages it is feeding you are captivating and convincing, borne out of your past experiences, but you must not allow yourself to be drawn in, you must quickly do something active, to engage the TPN.

Once you engage the TPN, you can usually turn the Demon back into the Angel it was before. You can redirect the imagination to feed the TPN with positive, constructive material. Then the DMN becomes the Angel it's meant to be: facilitative imagination. It's only when it is at rest, in repose, not creating, that it spews bile and becomes the Demon. When it feeds on itself, the angelic imagination turns demonic. This devil does indeed find work for idle hands.

One caveat: Even though we've touted the TPN as your ally and friend, it's important to note that it's not blameless and it, too, can go to the extreme. Indeed, we often refer to people who are the opposite of ADHD as having "attention surplus disorder." These are the bureaucrats, the automatons, the emotionless, by-the-book, detail-oriented types who are never late and always obey rules but never have new ideas and never laugh. They are habitually stuck in the TPN. Think about Uncle Ron and his analytical focus on his plants, losing sight of any empathy for the beloved wife he left at the store. When you're stuck in the TPN, it's easy to think about people in mechanical rather than relational ways. Whoever came up with the expression "one track mind" was inadvertently describing the TPN.

One study of managers showed that leaders totally focused on task are less supportive and nurturing of their teams than other managers. They can be rigid, narrow-minded, and unaccepting of ideas from others. Research suggests a quick fix is oxytocin, also known as the love drug or cuddle hormone, as it is released with a hug or warm social bonding. While a hug might not be appropriate in the workplace, it is something you can certainly try with a loved one. And for those with pets, you have a built-in prescription. Maybe it's time to bring more pets into the workplace!

WHAT CAN HANK DO?

If Hank could learn that the recurring thoughts and feelings that so torment him were not representations of dismal truth but artifacts of his prolific imagination, then he could learn to switch his focus away from those surges of fear and imagined doom that so haunt him and hold him back.

Perhaps Hank needs medication as well, but someone in his predicament is ripe for coaching on how to shut down the DMN, how not to feed the Demon. In finding ways of engaging his imagination in constructive tasks, he will be able to turn the DMN into an Angel, by connecting it—his imagination—to a useful task, thus activating the TPN. Meditation, exercise, and human connection can also reduce the power of the glitchy switches.

We have found this to be a monumentally useful insight for many of our patients. It's all new to them, hot off the presses of the scientific literature, ready to be used to put down the agonies the DMN can stir up.

While complicated in its anatomy, physiology, biochemistry, and synaptic flow, the DMN is easy to understand for the layman, if spelled out in plain English. So, as we recap, we'll keep it simple:

Don't feed the Demon.
Shut off its oxygen by denying it your attention.
Do something else that engages your mind.
Stay in action!

|

CHAPTER 3

The Cerebellum Connection

As our discussion of the TPN and DMN in the last chapter should make clear, we live in an era of increased understanding about the most dazzling, complicated, stupefying, powerful, protean, mystifying, and above all productive creation in all of nature: the human brain. And each of us gets to have one to call our very own!

A few numbers you might want to know about your brain: Far from physically beautiful to behold, weighing in at around 3 pounds (only about one-third the weight of a sperm whale's brain but about 15,000 times heavier than a goldfish's), the adult human brain houses about 100 billion cells. (Our own galaxy, the Milky Way, interestingly enough, contains about 100 billion stars.) Since each neuron connects with a hundred to thousands of other neurons at junctions called *synapses,* a staggering 150 trillion synapses enliven your brain and mine.

But on with our story. Another important brain-related development with huge and hopeful implications for people with ADHD or symptoms of VAST is our understanding of the area of the brain called the *cerebellum.*

Located at the base and back of the brain in two kumquat-shaped lobes, the cerebellum is small—it occupies only 10 percent of brain volume—but it is powerful: it contains a full 75 percent of the neurons of the brain.

We've known about the existence of the cerebellum for centuries—the Italian Renaissance artist Leonardo da Vinci used the term in his writing—and we've known that in concert with the vestibular system of the inner ear, it operates like a little gyroscope to coordinate our balance and physical movements. Indeed, the combined components are commonly referred to as the *vestibulocerebellar system,* or VCS, which is much less of a mouthful. The VCS is also implicated in the coordination and strengthening of various physical skills.

INNER WORKINGS (VCS BASICS)

That a fish is able to unconsciously and automatically maintain or change its place in the water is thanks to its VCS, always hard at work keeping the fish balanced and "aware" of whether it is moving vertically, horizontally, or diagonally.

This same orientation system has evolved—we're talking millions of years, as fish predate us—in humans, but in a far more sophisticated fashion. In fact, it's so sophisticated that it takes several years after birth before the human cerebellum and vestibular system reach maturity.

You can easily see how immature and poorly developed the human cerebellum is early on in life when watching a baby learn to walk. When babies start out, they stagger like drunks, only adorably so. But boy oh boy, just as toddlers do, our VCS comes on like gangbusters once it gets growing and helps us master new physical skills.

Or take the example of learning to ride a bike. At first, almost everyone has trouble finding their balance and coordinating the many small muscle movements needed to control wobbling and avoid falling. But gradually you learn to make the minute corrections that maintain your balance. Your VCS connects with your motor neurons, you lean a little this way or that, then voilà! You are soon off and cycling. (If you had to rely on your frontal cortex—the front, cortical part of the brain where we do our critical thinking—to calculate those corrections, you'd fall every time, because frontocortical thinking is about a hundred thousand times slower than the cerebellum's calculations.)

After some practice—longer for some, shorter for others—riding a bicycle becomes automatic, the neurologically necessary process ingrained. If you don't ride a bike for a while and feel kind of rusty when you try again, the VCS will help you steady yourself. But the pathways the cerebellum lays down tend to last. Once you learn to ride a bike, you can stay off bikes for decades only to get on again and ride off with hardly a quiver. Hence the expression "It's like riding a bike" to describe a skill you need to learn only once to have learned for life.

Anyone deeply engaged in an endeavor that requires split-second decisions out of nowhere is relying on the vestibulocerebellar system to kick in: a concert pianist, a brain surgeon, an airline pilot in an emergency landing. But consider the colorful and more visible (to the television audience, anyway) example of a football quarterback in action. Physical balance clearly matters, as he must run around ducking tacklers and avoiding sacks while also looking down the field. Keeping his balance is job one. But then there's so much more. If you were to list *all* the observations and calculations—and decisions based upon those observations and calculations—that the quarterback must make, the list would be hundreds of items long. And just exactly how much time does the quarterback get to do this? It is generally accepted that a pro quarterback must do something with the ball—throw a pass, hand the ball off, or run with it himself—within 2.8 seconds after the center snaps it to him. After 2.8 seconds, bad stuff happens. A sack, an interception, a fumble, a broken play.

Clearly, a quarterback does not have time to sit down with a protractor and a calculator and plot out his throw. He doesn't even have time to consciously flip through his memory bank of similar situations and decide what to do. His decision, which we think of more as a supremely conditioned reflex than an actual decision, derives from countless hours of film study, practice reps, rehearsed situations, drills, and more practice, until—allowing for some on-the-spot innovation—the decision becomes all but automatic. This entire process—this cascade of brain bifurcation points and synaptic firings—comes under the purview of the magnificent, newly knighted cerebellum.

Of course, things can go wrong.

Try this: Touch the tip of your nose with your index finger and then touch that same finger to something about a foot in front of you (the wall or a book or piece of furniture). Now touch your fingertip to your nose again. If this all comes easily to you, you have your cerebellum to thank—it's in working order, discerning distance and the orientation in space of the things you want to touch. If you misjudge the distance to the wall and back again or touch a spot in space rather than your nose, you are demonstrating *dysmetria*, an impairment of spatial judgment that means you miss the mark—the literal translation is "wrong length"—and indicates a malfunction in your cerebellum. Usually caused by an injury (surgery, trauma, infection, stroke, or another brain "insult"), other physical symptoms of cerebellar dysfunction include losing your balance easily, staggering, or impaired gait.

IMPROVED CEREBELLAR FUNCTION = IMPROVED ADHD SYMPTOMS

In 1998, our understanding of the cerebellum took a revolutionary step forward, with big (though unexpected) implications for ADHD. Jeremy Schmahmann, a professor of neurology at Harvard Medical School and a doctor at Massachusetts General Hospital (and now the director of the Schmahmann Lab for Neuroanatomy and Cerebellar Neurobiology at MGH), published a paper in *Trends in Cognitive Sciences* based on research he had done testing and observing people with injuries of the cerebellum. The paper was called *Dysmetria of Thought*. In it—as might be expected from this paper's title—he suggested that dysfunction of the cerebellum could cause us to lose not only our physical balance, but also our emotional equilibrium. In other words, just as the cerebellum had long been known to act as a kind of gyroscope or balancer of gait and movement, he explained, "so does it regulate the speed, capacity, consistency, and appropriateness of cognition and emotional processes."

By showing that the cerebellum plays a critical and central role in a person's ability to learn new skills, regulate emotion, and sustain focus, Schmahmann overturned generations of received wisdom. Put simply, his thinking was an innovative extrapolation from what had long been known about the function of the cerebellum. His research posited a far grander and more central role for the two kumquats at the back of the brain.

In fact, there is a now a well-recognized syndrome in neurology called *cerebellar cognitive affective syndrome* (CCAS) or, eponymously, simply Schmahmann's syndrome. It results from damage done to the cerebellum through stroke, trauma, surgical resection of a tumor, genetic anomaly, or any other insult. The symptoms of CCAS include problems with executive function, problems with linguistic processing, difficulty with spatial cognition (as assessed by drawing a clock or a cube), and affective (emotional) regulation. Does that list of cognitive issues sound familiar? Pretty darn close to ADHD.

In another paper (published in the *Journal of Neuropsychiatry and Clinical Neurosciences* in 2004), Schmahmann introduced the idea of a *universal cerebellar transform* (UCT) that acts as a stabilizer of thinking, emotion, and behavior. He called the UCT an "oscillation dampener," which means it works to diminish the erratic fluctuations in our thinking, feeling, and behavior. Using case studies of people in whom the UCT had been damaged, he described it as capable of automatically "smoothing out performance in all domains" without interrupting conscious thought, much as it does for the bicycle rider. And it helps you maintain what Schmahmann called a "homeostatic baseline," helping to preserve emotional and cognitive stability by sending out small signals that do not rise to the level of consciousness. This explains, at least in part, how you can guide a thought through a series of revisions, interruptions, or challenges in your mind without getting confused. It also helps explain how you can reach a fever pitch in a declaration of love without becoming psychotic, or how you can sustain anger without becoming incoherent. In a number of his injured or impaired patients, these capabilities were absent.

As mentioned earlier, one way to think about the central challenge in ADHD is gaining better braking control over the metaphorical Ferrari brain, both in terms of the speed at which it operates and the level of emotion it can emit. If Schmahmann's research proves that cerebellar injuries of all kinds can lead to the loss of control of the oscillation dampener (the brakes), it's not a big leap to postulate that by beefing up or returning the cerebellum to top working order, you might beef up your braking power, enhancing control over thought and emotion without losing any talents or capabilities in the process.

Based on Schmahmann's research, and based on the findings from other MRI studies that show that the central strip down the midline of the cerebellum—called the *vermis*—is ever so slightly smaller in people who have ADHD than in people who do not,[*1] it makes sense to think that stimulating and challenging the cerebellum/VCS, the way lifting a weight stimulates and challenges a muscle, might help reduce the negative symptoms of ADHD. This idea gets a major assist from neuroplasticity, the concept that the brain can change over a lifetime (discussed in chapter 2). Among all the regions of the brain, the cerebellum is the most plastic, the most changeable of all, able to promote the growth of existing neurons, making them look, on scans, bushier, with more interconnecting branches, like full treetops. Basically, it's been shown that you can take your cerebellum to the cerebellar gym and beef it up.

And that's exactly what a number of current treatments aim to do.

NEW TREATMENTS IN THE BALANCE

An obvious way to improve vestibular health and possibly increase cerebellar strength is to work on one's balance. And, in fact, the idea that using balancing exercises can help ADHD (and dyslexia) has been in the air for decades. In the 1960s a man named Frank Belgau invented the Belgau Balance Board. Based on his empirical observation that balance and learning go hand in hand (a special educator in Houston, Belgau had major learning problems himself[*2]), Belgau developed his balance board treatment to help his students. He never did the controlled studies needed to make the treatment scientifically legitimate and gain commercial momentum, but Mr. Belgau has many devotees and believers—his boards are still marketed and available today under the auspices of a company called Learning Breakthrough.

A trained chiropractor named Robert Melillo has taken Mr. Belgau's work one step further, writing a book entitled *Disconnected Kids*. Based on that work, he created a corporation that franchised over one hundred Brain Balance Achievement Centers around the United States. The balancing exercise protocols developed and offered at these centers work off Melillo's ideas about connection and disconnection between the hemispheres of the brain. Mr. Melillo's brain balance program is aimed at kids with more severe conditions than run-of-the-mill ADHD. You have to go to the center three times per week for one hour, so, including travel, the time commitment is high. And, depending on the center, the fees are not low. However, in our opinion, they do provide a valuable and usually successful treatment for selected children with more severe ADHD or autism.

Another program worth mentioning that is useful for a wide range of issues—from spatial awareness to learning issues—is called Zing Performance. Dr. Hallowell's son used Zing techniques for a reading problem, and his wife enrolled because she had the habit of driving over curbs! Both were greatly helped by the process.

In Zing, the subject first goes through a physical assessment of eye tracking speed and accuracy as well as attention span, either in person or online. Once the assessment is complete, the subject gets a series of exercises to do for ten minutes, twice a day. Zing has a wide repertoire of exercises that vary in practice but that all stimulate the cerebellum and the vestibular system through challenging balance and coordination.

The exercises include rotational stimulation, which has you turn around and around, the way you did as a kid, to make yourself dizzy, thus activating the vestibular system. Or lateral stimulation, which includes tilting from side to side with variations on that theme. And then vertical stimulation, which includes jumping and hopping in place or hopping forward.

You may be asked to stand on a wobble board not unlike those developed by Mr. Belgau. Once you get good at that, you're asked to stand on the board with your eyes closed. And then, still with eyes closed, to do some simple arithmetic calculations or repeat a series of numbers backward. Once you open your eyes, you're asked to toss a ball, then two balls, up in the air and catch them while you're still on the wobble board.

Regardless of the specifics, the exercises increase in difficulty as the subject progresses through the program, which typically takes three to six months. But, no pain, no gain! And the gain is clear. These exercises, if done faithfully, do indeed work the vestibular system hard, and many report subsequent improvements in the symptoms of ADHD.

Zing is working on getting the funding and organization for a randomized controlled trial, which would be the gold-standard test of its efficacy. In the meantime, Zing does have some impressive numbers to support the method. Fifty thousand people (of all ages) have gone through the Zing program for treatment of ADHD and/or dyslexia. According to Wynford Dore, Zing's founder, 80 percent achieve significant success. Dore himself is so confident in the treatment that he offers a money-back guarantee to all who sign up for the program; he reports that he is very rarely asked for refunds. (To learn more, and to see Dr. Hallowell's interview with Wynford Dore, go to distraction.zingperformance.com.)

A personal aside: We have seen so many possible breakthroughs fizzle that we've become a little jaded. We've learned the wisdom in the saying "When a new and exciting treatment for anything comes along, hurry to use it as soon as you can, while it still works." We've seen quite a number of treatments, from new drugs to new devices and brain games, go from being the greatest thing since sliced bread to being about as valuable as a single slice of that bread. Dr. Hallowell, however, has been offering the Zing treatment to some of his patients with good results. At the very least it is another tool in our toolbox, and a potential game changer.

THE INNER EAR AND ONE OUTSIDE-THE-BOX DOCTOR

More than twenty years before Dr. Schmahmann published his work on the sensitivities of the cerebellum and the workings of the inner ear, one pioneering—or off-the-tracks, depending on your point of view—doctor began working successfully with treatments for ADHD (and dyslexia) that Dr. Schmahmann's research might begin to explain. The pioneer in question is Harold Levinson, M.D., and (at this writing) he's practicing today, though he is still very much considered out of the mainstream. His treatment protocol has been to prescribe motion sickness medications like meclizine (Antivert, Bonine), Dramamine, and more recently the marvelously flexible Benadryl to people with ADHD and dyslexia. We admire Dr. Levinson for his courage in sticking to his guns, especially because he reports that his patients are getting excellent results. It's hard to believe they would have continued to come to him for decades were they not achieving at least some positive results from his unusual—but maybe no longer so crazy-sounding—regimen.

Now that it is becoming clearer that the inner ear and vestibular system play a significant role in ADHD, dyslexia, and an array of other conditions, Dr. Levinson may gain more respect. On the other hand, neither of us prescribes antihistamines or motion sickness medications for ADHD, dyslexia, or VAST because we have not seen or carefully studied the benefits ourselves. But we both agree with the mounting evidence that the vestibulocerebellar system is far more in play than we previously understood.

A CASE HISTORY

Dr. Hallowell recently made use of VCS stimulation in a fascinating but highly unusual consultation he did via email on a little boy in Shanghai. The story—related below by Dr. Hallowell—shows not only the power of working on one's balance, but also the other themes we emphasize throughout this book: the power of finding connection and focusing on strengths over weaknesses.

On a sunny Monday morning in October of 2018, I stood in the spacious pit of an amphitheater in Shanghai before an audience of some 250 Chinese adults, 90 percent female—mothers, teachers, and (as I came to find out later) a few grandmothers.

I've given thousands of presentations, but that day I was more nervous than I'd ever been before giving a talk. Having arrived in Shanghai the day before, I was at last about to find out if my ideas could pull their weight in China, a country with such a different culture from my country's, three thousand years of history compared to only about four hundred (since the 1607 settlement of Jamestown), a totally different language, four times as many people, and a form of government I'd read about all my life but still didn't understand.

At least I did understand ADHD. I'd long dreamed of bringing my approach across the Pacific to help the children in China, but I had no idea how the Chinese would receive it. Would my emphasis on the human connection fly? Would a country that still used corporal punishment in school be receptive to an American promoting the notion of helping children feel safe and secure in the classroom above all else? How would the Chinese take to my saying that since computers memorize better than humans, teachers ought to emphasize the development of the imagination in children instead of rote memorization? Might the whole concept of attentional and emotional problems be dismissed as disciplinary problems in disguise?

Within seconds I would find out. With my translator standing next to me, I took a deep breath and began to talk. I'd never done this before, speaking in short bursts, pausing for translation, before picking up where I left off, then pausing again. Also new to me: I had no notes, no slides, no script of any kind. The bulk of my talk described the behavior, diagnosis, and compassionate, strength-based treatment of a composite character, a boy whose characteristics and issues were made up to protect privacy but were wholly based on the real people in my practice.

At first I couldn't read the audience at all. These women were staring blankly back at me as if I were speaking, well, English, while they spoke only Chinese. But as the bursts of translation began to sink in, and I watched in silence as they listened to the translation, I could see the facial expressions in the audience change ever so slightly. But ever so slightly is all it takes when it comes to facial expressions. Millimeters tell all.

I began to feed off the energy of the audience and became increasingly animated. I could see them laughing—actually, tittering—at me slightly, but I could tell it was affectionate tittering. I also sensed that my ideas were resonating and sinking in. I could see some tears begin to trickle down cheeks as I panned the audience each time I paused for translation.

When the talk ended, I got huge applause, and a number of audience members came to the dais to meet me or to buy a copy of *Driven to Distraction,* which had been translated into Chinese.

One mother came up and stood nervously in front of me. After others had spoken, I noticed she still had not had her chance, holding back politely, so I invited her to speak. Thanking me, she told me how perfectly her seven-year-old son fit the description of the boy with attention problems that I described in my talk. As she described him it was all I could do to contain myself. "We *must* get him the help he needs," I said. "Right now." *But how?* I wondered.

Since the mother lived here in Shanghai, I suggested we email each other and try to work out a plan.

Over the following several months we did exactly that. What ensued was the most unusual case I've ever conducted in my forty-year career. I met the mother, whom I'll call Lily, in person only that one time, for about a minute. I never met the patient, her son—let's call him Samuel—at all.

But Lily was not deterred by these facts; she didn't feel that she could find the help she needed for Samuel in Shanghai. I asked her, via email, what could I do, seven thousand miles away, to help her son, not knowing her, him, his father, the school, the teacher, the language, the curriculum, the customs, the country, the resources, basically not knowing anything at all?

This is where my own ADHD and VAST characteristics came into play. The challenge energized me. This felt like the right kind of difficult for me (see chapter 5!). Lily wanted me to give it a try. I didn't think I could do any harm. So I said, via email, *Let's give it a shot.*

First, I had to take a history and make a diagnosis. Samuel was having trouble in school. Lily sent me a photo of him, showing a really cute little boy in blue shorts and a yellow shirt playing soccer outside. He looked cheerful, likable, and happy, but Lily told me about the trouble he was having focusing and remembering directions and how his grades were suffering. Samuel was becoming unhappier by the day.

Adding to his history was that he was left-handed and had been "corrected," as the Chinese put it, so now he was writing with his right hand. I knew that this kind of "correction" often causes its own problems.

Not knowing how Lily would receive it, or whether she would be able to make sense of it, I sent her the DSM-5 criteria for ADHD and asked her to check off all the symptoms that she felt applied to Samuel.

She replied immediately, less than twenty-four hours after I pushed Send on my email to her. In her opinion, Samuel had every single symptom listed in DSM-5. Had this been a traditional assessment, the diagnosis would be clear: ADHD, combined type.

Psychiatric treatment depends more than anything else, and more than in any other specialty, on the relationship between the patient and the doctor. While technically Samuel was the patient, practically speaking, Lily was; and she and I were off to a great start.

For all that we had going against us, on the plus side, Lily spoke and wrote good English, so my ignorance of Chinese would not matter much. In addition, she was highly motivated and had already demonstrated that she wanted to work with me to help her son.

But I had to ask myself whether I could devise a treatment plan that Lily could implement simply by following my suggestions via email. She did not have easy access to a psychiatrist, so there'd be no doctor in China involved, which meant we could not use medication.

You make do with what you've got. We were blessed to have email, which afforded speedy communication, as well as a massively motivated, intelligent mom, not to mention, as it turned out, a massively motivated, intelligent little boy.

This started to get fun, though it was a challenge, for sure. I put together a treatment plan based on the following elements:

1. My establishing trust with Lily.
2. Her having read *Driven to Distraction* in Chinese, enabling her to explain my background and recommendations to her husband, to Samuel, and to his teachers.
3. A strength-based model. Lily explained to Samuel that he had a race car for a brain, but with bicycle brakes. I told her it was key for him to understand that his race car brain was a great asset of which he should feel proud. He just needed to work on his brakes, so that then he could win races and become a champion.
4. Human connection and warmth. I asked Lily to hug Samuel a lot, in the morning and in the evening, and tell him how much she loved him. I stressed the importance of touch. Because he got so many reprimands at school, he needed to get lots of love at home. I also told her to ask the school to stop hitting him. If they were willing to put an end to corporal punishment, I was sure that Samuel would progress much more rapidly. My humble suggestion to the school was "Try treating him with kindness and warmth."
5. The promotion of a positive mindset. I asked Lily to adopt a constant

"You can do it" approach with Samuel, to try to implant in him the conviction that not only *could* he succeed but he *would* succeed.

6. Reading aloud to him each night.

7. Each day before school, Lily's telling him how much she loved him, what a fast brain he had, that all he needed to do was strengthen his brakes and he would win races, that one day he would be a champion and would bring great credit to his family and his country.

8. Having Samuel do balancing exercises (cerebellar stimulation). Samuel already played football (soccer), and he got plenty of traditional exercise. So I gave Lily a set of exercises that challenge balance and coordination. This was my homespun version of the Zing program as I explained it to Lily: Samuel should do the balancing exercises listed below for thirty minutes every day, in any order he wanted. I assured her that he could change them around for variety. If you can, I said, get a wobble board, a board with a rounded bottom so that it's hard to balance on. Also get an inflatable exercise ball that's big enough for him to sit on so his legs can't touch the floor.

   1. Stand on one leg for one minute or until he falls over.
   2. Stand on one leg with eyes closed for one minute or until he falls over.
   3. Take off socks and then put on socks without sitting down.
   4. Stand on wobble board for as long as he can, up to five minutes, then do it with eyes closed.
   5. Sit on exercise ball with feet off the floor for as long as he can, up to five minutes, then do it with eyes closed.
   6. Put five playing cards on the floor. Standing on one leg, bend over and pick up one card at a time.
   7. Do a low plank hold (elbows down on the ground, feet extended behind) for up to three minutes.
   8. Learn to juggle balls, and then spend three to five minutes juggling.

Samuel started doing the exercises right away, and Lily held up her end of the program as well. She hugged him, and she got her husband to do the same.

They changed their approach to talking with Samuel and asked his school to do so also. To help the cause, Lily shared our book with his main teacher, who in turn shared it with her administrators. Once Samuel started to improve, they agreed to stop corporal punishments.

To hear Lily tell it, Samuel started to improve within a matter of weeks—noticeably so. He was doing better in school—more focused, less disruptive of his classes, more successful with homework and class participation. The news of his transformation seemed to spread, she said, like juicy gossip. Parents wanted to know what was going on with Samuel. Why were his scores going up so much? They asked Lily what she was doing differently. No more yelling, no more hitting, she explained. Many were surprised that Lily's husband was going along with this plan, but no one seemed to be arguing with the results: Samuel's better behavior and greater happiness. Lily reported that others seemed impressed. All of this happened in a few short weeks, and it continued for months.

Connection. Education. Exercise with an emphasis on cerebellar stimulation. A strength-based model.

One day Samuel was given a chocolate for being the top student on a Chinese exam. He brought the chocolate home and gave it to Lily. She asked him, "Would you like to eat this now?"

He said, "Oh, no, Mom. That chocolate is much too important to eat."

The first key element to this success story was connection. Making the connection in person with Mom through my lecture was crucial. Even though I didn't speak Chinese, Lily spoke English, and we relied on help from translation software to fill in the blanks. The information I provided opened Lily's eyes; it was an "Aha!" moment. Suddenly she could see what was going on with Samuel. He wasn't lazy. He didn't need punishments and beatings. He needed to learn how to control his race car brain. Lily was mentally agile enough herself to "get it" right away, and to run with it.

Once we had made the connection and established trust, the next key element was education. Getting both parents and several teachers on board so fast was, by comparison to what I've had to do in the United States, breathtaking. Based on what I'd been told before going to China, I would have expected the opposite.

But then creating the right environment, the stellar environment, at school was crucial. That the school was willing to do everything I suggested reflects so very well on that school. Samuel would never have achieved the success he did without that.

It was also important that they understood the "race car brain with bicycle brakes" model of ADHD, because it is accurate but not shaming. It allowed Samuel to aspire to become a champion if he worked on his brakes, but it reminded him that there was work to be done. The key here was to use the model consistently. Instead of saying "You're a bad boy!" or "Shape up!" Lily said, "Your brakes are failing you." She still intervened, making it clear that certain behaviors needed to stop or change, but she did not do this via shame. This is critical to the long-term growth and success of the child. Shame is the most disabling learning disability.

The cerebellar exercises were the main, indeed the only, strictly therapeutic intervention I used with Samuel. They worked wonders. In all honesty, I was amazed to see how rapidly he progressed. Now, nearly three years later, I'm still in touch with Lily. She tells me the progress continues, and Samuel is thriving.

How much did all this mean to him? So much that chocolate became too precious to eat. I can't imagine a seven-year-old expressing pride more ardently than that.

SKIP NOTES

*1 The difference is not so big as to contribute to a diagnostic test, but it's a big enough difference, in large group aggregates of MRIs, to be significant and worthy of further study.

*2 Full disclosure: Dr. Hallowell wrote the introduction to Belgau's memoir about his life's work, *A Life in Balance*.

CHAPTER 4

The Healing Power of Connection

In 1985, Dr. Vincent Felitti, then chief of preventive medicine at Kaiser Permanente in San Diego, was running an obesity clinic for women and getting pretty good results. However, he kept seeing a recurring phenomenon he couldn't explain. A large number of patients who were doing well would drop out short of their goal, despite having started to successfully lose weight. A woman who needed to lose 300 pounds would lose 100 of those pounds but then, for no apparent reason or given explanation, abruptly drop out of the program.

A naturally curious man, Dr. Felitti decided to interview these women in more detail. He needed to know what was going on. One of the questions he asked in this deeper dive was "How old were you when you had your first sexual experience?" However, one day, tired from so many interviews, Dr. Felitti misspoke and asked one woman what he thought was a ridiculous question the minute it left his lips: "How much did you weigh when you had your first sexual experience?" It turned out instead to be the most important question he ever asked; it made medical history.

To Felitti's surprise, the woman did not find the question ridiculous at all. Painful in the extreme, to be sure, but not ridiculous. "Forty pounds. I was four years old and it was with my father," she replied, and then she burst into tears.

This was only the second case of incest Dr. Felitti had ever encountered, so he didn't expect to encounter many more. But he was intrigued by the possible connection between trauma and weight management so he added this question to his regular interview script. The more women he asked, the more common were reports not only of incest but of an array of other kinds of sexual abuse in their histories.

It turned out that many women dropped out of Dr. Felitti's weight loss program because losing weight made them feel unbearably anxious and vulnerable. Their girth helped them to feel safe, beyond a man's desire to assault them. So, even though they knew that their obesity put them at risk for disease, they did not want to give up the protection they felt it afforded them.

Felitti's accidental discovery led to a landmark study, one of the largest and most important public health surveys ever undertaken. Between 1995 and 1997, researchers interviewed some seventeen thousand subjects, all in the Kaiser Permanente HMO. These were largely white, upper-middle-class, college-educated San Diegoans who had good doctors, so the findings could not be attributed to poverty or lack of access to top-notch medical care. The researchers asked ten probing questions about incidents of emotional or physical trauma or abuse (including witnessing something traumatic or being the victim of it), exposure to drug or alcohol use (that is, being in the presence of an adult who abused these substances), and familial mental health. The results were startling: Two-thirds reported one experience on what's come to be called the Adverse Childhood Experience Scale, or ACEs. Twenty percent reported three or more experiences, and 13 percent reported four or more.

Since that initial finding, the Centers for Disease Control has continued this study, and the ACEs test has become a standard screening tool in many medical practices. That's because it can predict problems in adult health, both physical and mental: A score of four or more correlates with a 390 percent increase in chronic pulmonary disease; a 240 percent increase in liver disease; a 460 percent increase in depression; and a 1,220 percent increase in suicide attempts. Even a score of one correlates with a marked increase in adult alcoholism, depression, and divorce.

Dr. Vivek Murthy, the nineteenth Surgeon General of the United States and author of the book *Together: The Healing Power of Connection in a*

Sometimes Lonely World, named another adverse condition—loneliness—the number one medical problem in the country. In a *Harvard Business Review* essay, he said:

> During my years caring for patients, the most common pathology I saw was not heart disease or diabetes; it was loneliness. Loneliness and weak social connections are associated with a reduction in lifespan similar to that caused by smoking fifteen cigarettes a day and even greater than that associated with obesity. Loneliness is also associated with a greater risk of cardiovascular disease, dementia, depression, and anxiety. At work, loneliness reduces task performance, limits creativity, and impairs other aspects of executive function such as reasoning and decision making. For our health and our work, it is imperative that we address the loneliness epidemic quickly.

Why this matters so much in our story of ADHD is because, as you probably can guess, ACEs scores run much higher in families where there is ADHD, either in a parent or in a child, or both. Because the negative side of ADHD, the bad brakes, causes impulsive behavior often out of control, the parent is more likely to mistreat or abuse his child, and the child is more likely to provoke, alienate, or assault his parent. It's a dangerous setup on both sides, parent and child.

LOVE HEALS

If there was ever any doubt, the ACEs study proves once and for all that bad stuff in childhood—abuse, neglect, violence, drug use, loneliness, poverty, chaos—begets *really* bad stuff in adulthood. But there is an equally clear antidote. Connection, positive connection, which at its most distilled is called love, has incredible healing power.

The Columbia University professor and psychiatrist Kelli Harding gathered much of the research into the power of love and connection in her 2019 book, *The Rabbit Effect.* The title derives from a study on rabbits who were fed a high-fat diet to show the effect of high cholesterol on the health of the heart. Not surprisingly, the rabbits showed large deposits of fat in their coronary arteries on autopsy. They had not been healthy.

Except for one anomalous group of rabbits that showed 60 percent fewer fatty deposits than all the others. Same diet, same strain of rabbits, same lab, same age, but this one group had markedly lower deposits of fat in their hearts. It was a complete mystery to the investigators.

Being good scientists, they looked further for an explanation. The salient variable that ended up explaining the difference had nothing to do with diet, exercise, genetics, or any of the other standard reasons a scientist might expect.

The explanation lay in the kindness shown to those rabbits by the lab technician who managed their group. She handled the rabbits in her care affectionately, talking to them and petting them while she fed them and cleaned their cages. She doted on them as a loving owner dotes on favorite pets. She was no mere lab tech, she was a purveyor of love. Love made the difference.

In humans, a famous research project known as the Grant Study—in which researchers from Harvard Medical School studied 268 Harvard College sophomores from the classes of 1939 through 1944 and followed them for the rest of their lives—was brought to prominence by Harvard's George Vaillant through his forty years of monitoring the study. Under a new lead researcher, Harvard psychiatrist Robert Waldinger, the study is still under way today, making it the longest-running longitudinal study of adult development ever done. Its main conclusion is beautifully and compellingly simple. The single most important factor in predicting health, longevity, occupational success, income, leadership ability, and general happiness comes down to one four-letter word. "It's love," Vaillant famously stated. "Full stop."

In his summary of the Grant Study findings, published in *Triumphs of Experience: The Men of the Harvard Grant Study,* Vaillant wrote about one of the most important lessons from the study, that in order for love to work its most sustaining magic, the individual who is loved must be able to receive the love, to metabolize it, to use Vaillant's word. Even if you had a loveless childhood and feel empty at age twenty-five, by age seventy-five you can feel fulfilled and content if you've learned how to take love in rather than push it away.

Dr. Hallowell can personally attest to the truth of Vaillant's finding. His ACEs score is eight. Given the increased risks for a score as low as four, an eight obviously puts him at great risk. He ought to be alienated from his children, depressed, alcoholic, out of work, lonely and sick, and near death's door.

Instead, he has enjoyed more than thirty-three happy years of marriage and raised three well-adjusted and treasured children; he is seventy-one healthy years old at this writing.

Statistically speaking, Dr. Hallowell is an outlier: He has beaten extreme odds. But he knows why he beat the odds, and he knows why almost every person like him beats the odds: the unsurpassed power of positive connection —Vitamin Connect, or, as we like to say, "the other vitamin C." In his case, he had a particularly loving and magical connection with his grandmother, whom he called Gammy. Aware of his hardships and sensitive to his needs, she seemed to make it her mission to give him safe haven. Their time together was both memorable and precious. As he puts it:

> Gammy could turn peeling a hardboiled egg into a surgical search for a Golden Kingdom called Yolk. She could turn a rainy day into a festival, a croquet mallet into a Queen's scepter. She could take a disappointed boy, upset by unkind words from a friend, and turn that boy into a barrel of laughs in two shakes of a lamb's tail, to use one of her favorite expressions. She could elevate the lowliest day to the heights of delight. A visit to Gammy's took on an electric charge the moment it was announced.

FEELING UNDERSTOOD

Creating comfortable, positively connected environments is the most important step in helping people of all ages get the most out of life in general; the lack of connection particularly hurts people who have ADHD.

In his book *The Globalization of Addiction*, Bruce Alexander uses the term "dislocation" (which was coined by the political economist Karl Polanyi) to refer to the loss of "psychosocial integration." Dislocation, he explains, is psychologically toxic and untenable. An individual will crack in any number of ways: disruptive behavior; extreme anxiety; withdrawal; school refusal; the beginnings of substance use; depression and thoughts of suicide; the development of an eating disorder; cutting; poor performance at work; loss of job; marital difficulties. The dismal list goes on.

While Alexander's focus is on addiction—of all kinds, including addiction to screens—his words perfectly describe how many children with ADHD feel in classrooms and adults with ADHD feel in the adult world. Misunderstood, alienated, left out, on the outside looking in.

Sometimes literally on the outside. Dav Pilkey, the writer and illustrator who created the beloved Captain Underpants series of books (and many other children's books), spent most of his elementary school years sitting alone outside in the hallway after being paddled with a board by the principal. How terrible it is that millions of children with ADHD suffer similarly from the lack of sustaining connection simply because they are different, because their minds run like race cars with bad brakes, and because others fail to understand. Those of us with ADHD are usually pretty sensitive, so we begin to put up defenses, and before you know it we're loners, being teased, put off, or, if we're adults, not climbing the ladder, and people are wondering why, and not in a helpful way.

The experience of living with this condition is like being part of an invisible minority. Even if you do become visible, even if you do get identified and treated, you usually still face prejudice: "Oh, he's a Special Ed kid." "He's a *re*tard." "He's got ADHD, whatever that is." "He takes Adderall." The stigma rules.

What we need—especially as children—is not punishment or ridicule; what we need is free and easy to supply—Vitamin Connect. Without it, we feel more and more separate, alone, and apart. "Psychosocial integration" may be a cumbersome term, but it connotes a warm and wonderful force everyone can understand and every child and every adult in every organization ought to get many doses of every day. It should be the lifeblood of all families, schools, and organizations.

Peter, as we'll call him, is typical of the patients we see in our consulting practices, and the outline of his story points up the tremendous importance of connection. When he was sixteen and in tenth grade, he came to Dr. Hallowell's office with his parents. By all accounts—his parents' and his teachers'—he was very smart and hugely talented, but he had trouble finishing assignments, so his grades didn't show it. He felt his teachers were often well-meaning, but he also felt beaten down from the effort of toeing the line all the time at school. He believed he was "stupid," and he generally lacked motivation for the school he had come to hate. Were it not for his likely-ADHD pediatrician father and his smart neuroscientist mom, he would have been a candidate for residential treatment. They believed in their son and stayed connected with him as they tried to help him find his way.

As Peter discussed with Dr. Hallowell what really interested him, it became clear that he was happiest when making things out of wood. The family hatched a plan: Peter would go to the local vocational tech school in his area for eleventh grade, and Peter's father agreed to set up a woodworking shop in their basement so that Peter could explore that talent fully. There were other strategies, too—he tried cerebellar stimulation treatment (see chapter 3), and he and Dr. Hallowell discussed the nature of the brain's default mode network (see chapter 2) and how it was contributing to Peter's brooding and rumination. Lastly, Dr. Hallowell prescribed the use of a medication off-label (Amantadine—see chapter 8), which he believed could help Peter when the other meds he'd tried hadn't. Dr. Hallowell made clear that the road ahead would not be smooth for Peter, but with his parents' belief in him, and now a warm connection with Dr. Hallowell, Peter reported to his mother (who later reported it to Dr. Hallowell) that he was at last feeling understood, and for the first time in the longest while, feeling hopeful.

In first grade, one amazing teacher gave her understanding—a powerful antidote to dislocation—to Dr. Hallowell himself:

In first grade I couldn't read. At reading period we'd take turns reading out loud, "See Spot run, run, run, run, up, up, up, down, down, down." Simple. But I couldn't read that. I had dyslexia. Back then, unless you had a wise teacher, you were called *slow,* which meant stupid, and so they skipped you when it was your turn to read. But my teacher, Mrs. Eldredge, was wise. She didn't skip me. She'd just come over and sit down next to me when it was my turn to read, and she'd put her arm around me and pull me in close to her. As I would stammer and stutter through "up, up, up," none of the kids would laugh at me because I had the mafia sitting next to me. Mrs. Eldredge's arm was my treatment plan. She gave me psychosocial integration. Every day.

It was brilliant. It was all she could do—she couldn't cure my dyslexia and they didn't have an Orton-Gillingham tutor* in the school —but it was all she needed to do. With that arm—with the power of connection—she cured the real learning disabilities, which are fear, and shame, and believing that you can't do something. To this day I am a painfully slow reader—my wife teasingly says she can't believe I know *anything*—but I read well enough to have majored in English at Harvard, to have graduated with high honors, and to make part of my living now by writing books, none of which would have happened without Mrs. Eldredge and the loving connection her arm gave me.

We know all too well that you sink without enough connection, no matter how unsinkable you may think you are. Too many people don't tap into the power of connection nearly as much as they should because they claim to be too busy for connection, or they trivialize its power. But the deeper reason that some people avoid connection is that they fear it. They fear it because they've connected before and been hurt in a way they never want to be hurt again.

We say to them, and maybe to you, *Take heart.* Hearts heal. Unlike the ship synonymous with sinking, the titanic power of connection rises up from the deep every time it sinks, as long as we are brave enough to board her again. Once she knows we are ready to jump on, she rises, ready to welcome us once more.

We ought, all of us, to tap more often into the power of connection. Multitudinous science supports doing so. It only makes sense. How would you feel if you were criticized all day long, as so many of these children are? Fear is the major learning disability, fear and shame. We humans ignore connection until we nearly perish due to its absence. We are living in a massive Vitamin Connect deficiency.

TIPS FOR A RICHLY CONNECTED LIFE

Create for your child, for yourself, for your family, for your organization, for your community, for this country, and for this world if you possibly can, a connected life. It is the key to pretty much everything good in life. And it is, for the most part, free.

It's how to keep a bad childhood from ruining your life. Even better, developing positive connections is the best way to prevent a bad childhood.

Kindness makes kids grow, and adults as well. A deeply, variously connected life is the most enriching gift you can give yourself and your family. Connection comes in many forms. Here are more ideas—some pretty obvious and others a little off-the-wall—for using the amazing power of connection in your life or your child's. Add to this list in your own off-the-wall ways:

- Make a point of having meals with your family—family dinners have been proven to work wonders, even to improve SAT scores—and have meals with other people you know. It's wonderful to introduce children to people from out of town, even from out of the country, and make dinner a big deal where people meet to eat and greet. The more you do this, the more meals turn into events that take on meaning beyond merely a chance to refuel.

- Unless you or someone in your family is allergic, or your physical layout makes it impossible, get a pet! We are biased toward man's best friend—dogs—because of their companionability and their obvious, freely given love for their owners. But a cat, guinea pig, parrot, hamster, ferret, turtle, fish, or even a snake provides both a focus of our love and a sense of it in return. Pets give us "the other vitamin C" as no other being can.

- Make a daily stop at a favorite coffee shop with hellos all around. And get into the habit of giving hellos and nods to people you don't know. This kind of passing acknowledgment gives a quick dose of Vitamin Connect, and it prods you out of the habit of anonymity most of us slip into.

- Do the same thing at your favorite gas station. Of course, first you'll have to designate a favorite gas station and frequent it. But just imagine how much more fun it will be to fill up your car instead of dreading the cost and the lame feeling you have standing there pumping your gas, wondering whether this is all there is to life. If you actually knew the people at the station and you talked with them and turned the stop into a meaningful moment? Win-win!

- Keep up with at least two good friends regularly. This is even better than going to the gym every day! One way to do this is to have a standing lunch date or a time reserved for a catch-up phone call every week. Soon you will really look forward to this regular shot in the arm of love and familiarity.

- Plan a sleepover for your child. Or invite your own grandchild for the night. Having extended, agenda-free (except for play!) time with another young person (or *a* young person, if you're the grandparent) is hugely restorative and connective.

- Reserve at least a half hour of uninterrupted one-on-one time with your child every week, no agenda, doing whatever your child wants as long as it's safe, legal, and not too expensive. Child psychiatrist Dr. Peter Metz calls this "special time," and he says it works magic on the parent-child relationship and for a child's sense of belonging and love.

- Join some kind of group that holds meetings—a book club, a lecture series, a knitting circle. Then attend those meetings! The MacArthur Foundation Study on Aging showed this to be one of the two factors most associated with long life (the other is frequency of visits with friends).

- Clear yourself of pent-up anger and resentment—that is, practice forgiveness of others and of yourself. Do this as often as you fill up your car with gas. There is no one way to do this; you'll have to find a way that works for you. One example: You say to yourself, *He was a son of a bitch, but I am not going to waste one more second of my precious life being angry at him.* Forgiveness does not mean that you condone the deed, just that you renounce the hold that anger has over you.

- Take a daily inventory of gratitude. This sounds corny, but it feels really good. Whether you make a written list or just take the time to go over what you're grateful for in your mind, you come away feeling lighter and more optimistic.

- Make a point of paying compliments. This may feel awkward, but how much do you love it when someone notices and comments on something good about you? Give that kindness back and you will likewise feel good!

- Engage in some kind of spiritual practice, whether as an individual or in a group. It doesn't have to be organized religion, just some framework for entertaining and sharing the Big Questions, Ideas, Uncertainties, Possibilities, and Hopes. Finding the right group is key, but once you do find such a connection, it will reach into, enlighten, and warm many areas of your life.

- Go for a walk in nature alone or with a friend (and preferably with that dog we want you to adopt!).

- Never worry alone. This one is *key*. Of course, choose with care the people you worry with. But when you worry with the right person, worry quickly turns into a chance to problem-solve and sometimes even a chance to laugh—releasing your worries—together.

- Minimize your consumption of news if it tends to upset you or rile you up. If you feel more connected to the world through watching it, however, don't give it up!

- Visit graveyards—whether someone you love is interred there or not. Strolling around a cemetery can cast a special spell, making us feel reverent and quiet, and often strangely rejuvenated.

- Whatever you're wrestling with, take a bow for working so hard to be a better person. In other words, connect with your desire to improve and give yourself credit for trying to do that.

- Connect with your personal vision of greatness and try to hold it in your consciousness every day as a guide and inspiration. One way to do this is to identify one living person you admire, then allow that admiration to lift you up.

- Learn about your ancestors. You can do this either through archival research or asking questions of your elders. Asking questions has the added bonus of connecting you to those elders.

- Along the same lines, talk to non-related old people about their lives, in detail. This is like reading a great novel.

- Visit the local fire department if you can, and talk to a fireman about his job. Firemen love to talk, and they tend to be great connectors.

- Climb a tree and sit on a branch for at least ten minutes; it gives you a point of view on the world you rarely can achieve and, chances are, haven't seen since you were ten years old. Don't have a tree (or the ability to climb one)? Try sitting in the middle of a town square or on a bench along a busy walkway. You'll be amazed at who and what you see passing by if you spend the time to just observe. Doing this doesn't necessarily connect you to another individual, but rather to the humanity passing by.

- Associate with dream makers. Avoid dream breakers. Cynics may be funny and entertaining, but they tend to drain you of hope. As Oscar Wilde said, a cynic is one who "knows the price of everything, and the value of nothing."

- Always be on the lookout for the person who can provide for your child (or for you) what you can't.

- Be on the lookout for any charismatic mentor. Many studies show that charismatic mentors—not grades, study habits, where they go to school, or IQ—make the biggest difference in kids with ADHD and VAST. If they can find a teacher, coach, family friend, or anyone else who understands and inspires them, then the sky truly is the limit.

---

* Orton-Gillingham is a multisensory phonics approach to teaching reading.

CHAPTER 5

I

Find Your Right Difficult

Most people who have ADHD or VAST are naturally creative and original. They think along unusual lines and feel a persistent drive to build, develop, or create something, anything, from a business to a boat to a book to a balustrade. It's like an omnipresent itch to *make something.*

If that itch goes unscratched, we tend to feel listless or depressed, unmotivated and at sea. If we pour our energies into something that is beneath our creative abilities, we tend to lose interest. Remember, boredom = kryptonite. If we find ourselves in a job that doesn't draw on that creative strength but instead demands a skill set we just don't have, we will falter—and we'll feel the crush of that defeat harder than others do. But once we find an outlet for our creativity that is a Goldilocks kind of *just right,* once we find a project to sink our teeth into, then *presto!* we light up like a Christmas tree.

What's your outlet, your child's instrument, stage, or tool? What's your right kind of difficult?

TAPPING INTO SUPERPOWER

Being syndromes of matched opposite characteristics—with an upside to every perceived downside—ADHD and VAST are unique among conditions in the behavioral sciences. Not recognizing this fact is the chief reason the strengths associated with ADHD/VAST got ignored for so long: Doctors tend to look for pathology and focus on problem behaviors. Which is to say, they often ignore strengths.

Of course, it's true that most people who have ADHD or VAST are *really* bad at quite a few things (in which their noses get rubbed all the time), but usually they are, or could be, truly exceptional at one or two other activities. Toward that end, we take a strength-based approach to treating people in our practices. As we like to say, we do not treat disabilities, we help people unwrap their gifts. More exuberantly: We help identify superpowers!

Some people just luck into this outcome—one thing leads to another that reveals that superpower. To wit: Consider the journey of a man we'll call Allen. When he was in high school, Allen's motivation for getting a summer job was to have enough money to go on dates. He didn't have much patience for filling out the requisite job applications, though—a bugaboo for those of us with ADHD, to be sure—but luckily for him an opportunity fell in his lap. As it happened, a local rug cleaning company had a phone number one digit away from his family's phone number, so his house received a lot of wrong-number calls looking for the rug cleaning company. Instead of being annoyed at all the calls, the way most people would be, Allen's mind lit up. Only fourteen years old at the time, he saw a business opportunity. When a wrong-number call would come in, Allen would answer and say in his most charming, enthusiastic voice, "This is not the rug cleaning company you are looking for, but I can do a better job cleaning your rug than they can, and I will charge you a lower price!" He saw an opportunity where almost no one else would have, and he had the innate genius to grab it. It all happened in a flash, and before Allen knew it, he had himself a business.

Unfortunately, Allen wasn't old enough to drive (and he didn't have access to a car anyway), so he reached out to an older friend who had a car, and the two of them rented a rug cleaning machine. They'd go to the houses of the people who'd called the wrong number and accepted the invitation to try Allen's offer, and soon he and his partner were making $400 to $700, after expenses, every weekend, in 1975 dollars.

Allen continued to discover opportunities where others wouldn't see them. One day he was cleaning the rugs in a local professor's office when he noticed a piece of equipment stored there. Being naturally curious, as most people with ADHD or VAST tend to be, he asked what the equipment was for. It turned out that it was an old machine for editing film. On another visit to clean this professor's rugs, Allen saw someone cleaning the machine and asked if he could watch the process. When Allen saw that taking the machine apart, cleaning the lens, and reassembling it all was pretty simple, he decided to try to get into the film machinery cleaning field as well. This interest (and skill— turns out Allen could get the job done for $150 less than his competition!) led Allen to get a job with a local film production company and, in turn, to meet a number of well-known Bostonians, including the celebrity chef Julia Child and the famous Boston Celtic Larry Bird.

Wouldn't you know—at the time, the then governor of Massachusetts needed asbestos removed from a house he wanted to buy, and a realtor asked Allen about it, since Allen seemed to know a little something about cleaning all kinds of things. Rather than saying he didn't know (which would have been the truth), Allen took a three-day course on removing asbestos. He got a summer job with an asbestos removal company between eleventh and twelfth grades and removed the asbestos from the house the governor was to buy.

Allen worked hard at all these odd jobs, and people seemed to love his can-do, figure-it-out spirit. Soon he added still more skills to his résumé. At one point he met a family who owned a dog grooming business and went to work for them. Through dog grooming he met a number of wealthy people in the suburbs, one of whom ran an au pair company, and she hired Allen to be a tour guide for every new au pair that summer.

Allen is now in his fifties and a successful businessman in the asbestos removal sector. But he's still as creative and nimble as ever. He recently got his first patent approved, for a dustless dumpster system!

Allen's superpower is that he's a problem solver. And as long as he is intellectually challenged by the problem and is meeting interesting people and learning how things work, there's almost no one better at turning chance into opportunity.

Sometimes someone finds their superpower through this kind of serial entrepreneurship, but other times it might best be described as a kind of "lightning strike" of one particular interest. For instance, we know a professor at an Ivy League university whom we would identify as having VAST characteristics, if not diagnosed ADHD. When he was in college, he tells us, he couldn't find anything that interested him, so he seriously considered dropping out to become a ski bum.

Bags packed, he was ready to leave the small college he was attending when a girl he knew asked him to come to a physics lecture with her. He had absolutely no interest in physics—science basically bored him, especially compared to skiing—but he did like the girl, so he agreed to attend one last lecture before quitting college for good.

Less than a minute into the physics lecture he'd forgotten all about his date and was totally engrossed in the topic at hand. That one lecture opened up a torrent of interest, curiosity, and innate brilliance—a superpower—for a subject he had previously known nothing about. He went on to become one of the luminaries in the field.

Lightning like this does strike, and it isn't all that rare, either. We who have ADHD or VAST characteristics tend to fall in love in a hurry—with a person, with a subject, with a project, with a deal, with a plan. Sparks fly, and before you know it, we've forgotten how lost and forlorn we were because we're immersed in whatever it was that caught our attention.

But it's often the case that the identification of your superpower will take concerted effort, and perhaps some trial and error with challenges.

ASSESSING YOUR STRENGTHS

People with ADHD and VAST need a challenge. As we've said, boredom is our kryptonite. The trick, though, is not just to find a challenge—after all, digging a hole and filling it up is a challenge—but to find the *right* challenge. We call that *the right difficult.* One proactive way to pinpoint your right difficult is to develop a practical inventory of your strengths—what you are good at.

A simple way to start is to sit down with your child, or, if you're an adult, sit down with your spouse or some other adult (it's best to do this with another person, as the interaction makes for more creative, spontaneous, playful, and thorough answers), and respond to the following questions. Have the person asking the questions write down your answers, because this is an important document to save:

1. What three or four things are you best at doing?
2. What three or four things do you like doing the most?
3. What three or four activities or achievements have brought you the most praise in your life?
4. What are your three or four most cherished goals?
5. What three or four things would you most like to get better at?
6. What do others praise you for but you take for granted?
7. What, if anything, is easy for you but hard for others?
8. What do you spend a lot of time doing that you are really bad at?
9. What could your teacher or supervisor do so that your time could be spent more productively?
10. If you weren't afraid of getting in trouble, what would you tell your teacher or supervisor that he or she doesn't understand about you?

The answers to these ten questions reveal a lot. This information is gold. Armed with it, you can more productively talk with your child's teacher or your own employer to try to create a better learning or working environment.

If you are the parent of a child with ADHD or VAST characteristics, bring this brief assessment inventory to your child's school. Most of the time these children have files full of negative comments or failures. It's good to get positives into the record. It's also essential that the teacher know what your child's interests are—from dinosaurs to planets to sports to horses to videogames—so that he or she can come up with side projects to keep your child interested. This can be crucial, because a major reason kids with attention issues do poorly in school is that they feel bored, which in turn leads the teacher to believe they don't care about schoolwork. If the teacher can work your child's interests into the curriculum (or just allow your child to pursue them during downtime), your child is likely to show a whole new level of interest in school. This creates a positive feedback loop—your child's interest and attention in class may lead the teacher to more often give her or him the benefit of the doubt instead of assuming the worst or having a knee-jerk reaction to distracted behavior. The profile this short strengths assessment generates can also become part of your child's school file and be referred to by other teachers, specialists, and administrators when questions come up about their interests—or lack of interests—in future years.

For adults, this strengths assessment can be the starting point for looking for a new job or reevaluating your current one. As a guiding principle, you ought to spend the majority of your working hours at the intersection of three circles: the circle of all the things you really like to do, the circle of all the things you're really good at doing, and the circle of things that someone will pay you to do. You can use this strengths assessment to help you organize your thinking to find that intersection, that special zone where you ought to spend as much of your working day as you possibly can, because that's where you will do your best work and be happiest doing it.

GET TO KNOW YOUR STRENGTHS IN A WHOLE NEW WAY

Armed with awareness of your strengths, you're ready for the next test, one of the most powerful you can take, even if you've never heard of it: the Kolbe Index.

If you want to know what strengths you've always known you had but likely have never named, take this test. If you also want to know why some tasks have seemed all but impossible to you even though they come easily to others, take this test. If you want to know where your "sweet spot" is, where you ought to spend most of your time, in what kind of work, take this test.

The Kolbe test was developed by a brilliant and fearless pioneer named Kathy Kolbe. She'd grown up around test development—her father developed the Wonderlic Personnel Test (now known as the Wonderlic Contemporary Cognitive Ability Test), which is given to all incoming NFL players—but it wasn't until after graduating from Northwestern University that Kathy threw her own intellectual interest into figuring out why smart people aren't more productive or creative. She saw what IQ tests and other personality assessments didn't quite get at: that how a person exerts effort is defining. So she started work on an assessment tool that would unearth the unique and inborn way that each of us exerts effort or takes action. This, she reasoned, would show us a person's *conative* style. Stemming from the Latin word *conatus,* which means "effort," the dictionary definition of "conation" is "the mental faculty of purpose, desire, or will to perform an action; volition."

That's what Kathy wanted to investigate and assess, because after all, what are the strengths that matter most but the strengths that lead to action? Much more important than IQ, which is, from a practical standpoint, irrelevant, your conative style determines *what you actually do in life.* Borrowing again from the Latin, Kolbe calls this our MO, our *modus operandi.* And, for our purposes, *that's* what a person who has ADHD most needs to learn about herself or himself and why we so strongly recommend taking this test.

Over the years, Kolbe has developed her test and refined it, administering it to thousands upon thousands of individuals. It has now been validated in more than 1.6 million case studies over forty years.

Here's how Kathy explains it:

There's a part of the mind that you don't hear a lot about. It's what some people call "instincts" or that "gut feeling" when you're making a decision. Our secret: We know what natural strengths—instincts—you were born with, and how you can use those strengths to be the most productive, stress-free version of yourself.

There's *something already inside you that can rid the stress from your life,* help your relationships, and change the way you interact in the workplace. These strengths are proven to remain unchanging in long-term test-retest reliability studies.

If you're over sixteen, take the Kolbe A Index. If you're between ten and sixteen, look for the Kolbe Y Index.* Both of these trademarked tests are quick, easy, thirty-six-question assessments with no wrong answers. After you answer the questions, the test will generate a score comprised of four digits between one and ten. These numbers represent your innate aptitude in four areas of action, which Kolbe calls Fact Finder, Follow Thru, Quick Start, and

Implementor.

As an example of what these numbers mean, let's take a closer look at Dr. Hallowell's Kolbe Index score: 5, 3, 9, 2.

Dr. Hallowell's Fact Finder tendency score is 5. This relates to how he naturally gathers or shares information. Being a 5, he is right in the middle, what's called an *accommodator*. In other words, he tends to get all the facts *or* just go with a summary; consistently doing either one would be stressful for him. Most people with ADHD or VAST have low scores in Fact Finder (which does not mean bad; there are no bad scores on a Kolbe test) because their natural talent lies in their ability to cut to the chase and summarize information instead of digging into details.

Dr. Hallowell's Follow Thru score is 3. This denotes how he instinctively deals with the need for organization and processes. Being a 3, he is technically "resistant" in Follow Thru, which is typical of people with ADHD or VAST. In other words, they take shortcuts and let solutions evolve as they work on problems instead of planning an approach in advance.

Dr. Hallowell's Quick Start score is 9. This relates to how he approaches risk and uncertainty. With a 9 in Quick Start, he is "insistent" in this way, and that makes him like most people with ADHD or VAST. They jump right in without testing the waters first. Remember: fire, ready, aim.

The 2 in Dr. Hallowell's score refers to his Implementor tendencies, or how well he naturally deals with hands-on work and managing space. His score of 2 suggests that he *envisions* rather than arranges and physically protects the spaces in which he lives and works. Many people with ADHD or VAST are at the other end of this scale. They need to move and create movement as they work. They need to create physical, hand-built solutions to problems.

The Kolbe website explains this scoring system in detail, helping you make sense of where you stand and pointing you toward where you might focus your energies. As with anything worthwhile, you'll have to do some work to get the value. This is not a parlor trick. But the work you put in—we're talking a half hour to an hour—will pay off in a big way. Once you unlock the secrets those numbers contain, you will understand yourself in a much deeper and more helpful way.

Once you identify your strengths, using our short set of questions or taking the Kolbe test to learn about your MO, you're well on your way to the great prize of finding the right difficult.

NO, THANKS, DOC, I'LL TAKE THE *REALLY* HARD WAY (AKA WHAT'S UP WITH SELF-DEFEATING BEHAVIOR?)

It's a funny thing about those of us who have ADHD. We want what others avoid. We like problems. We *need* the difficult. That's because easy is boring. We need the stimulation of intense challenge. But as we've said, a challenge undertaken just for the sake of a challenge can be counterproductive at best, self-defeating at worst. As one patient—let's call him Jon—put it:

> What drives me is, unfortunately, not what makes me happy. A way to explain it is that the way my brain works is such that I constantly need to be working on impossibly difficult projects. If I'm not doing that, I get bored and restless. I told my wife that if you stuck me on a beach for a week and forced me to relax, and took away my iPhone and my pen and paper, after thirty minutes I'd start writing to-do lists and business ideas using my own blood. But that is not what makes me "happy" because such work is hard and stressful. So it's sort of a catch-22.
>
> Either I'm doing what drives me, which is intense problem solving every second I am awake, or I'm bored/anxious/don't know what to do with myself.

We hear explanations like Jon's all the time, heroic tales of someone grittily giving everything they've got in order to do what they find nearly impossible for reasons that have nothing to do with fame, money, or material gain. What drives this self-defeating narrative? A gut *need* to do the extremely difficult.

Because it's just not in the makeup of people with ADHD or VAST to give up. Sticking to something is a terrific quality if the something is productive and makes you happy or your life better. But sticking to something just for the sake of sticking to it is a Sisyphean undertaking—pushing that old boulder up the hill day after day only to have it roll back down the next. In some way, people like Jon seem almost to enjoy the process of perpetual failure, as if the real, hard truth of life is to be found in pain, suffering, and defeat. Their victory is to be found in carrying on no matter what.

To compound the problem, people with ADHD or VAST tendencies usually reject help. Of course, there is an upside to this trait—it's called nonconformity. Another, less polite way of saying it: People with attention issues tend to have acute bullshit detectors. We hate hypocrisy maybe more than any other human failing, and we can spot it a mile away. We don't join cults. That's definitely a positive side of rejecting help.

But taken to the extreme, this is counterproductive. Rejecting help can sabotage a person's education, career, health, and relationships. As we've stated earlier, it's not uncommon for a young person or adult to say, "I'd rather fail doing it my way than succeed with help." A patient we'll call Greg tried to explain his resistance to accepting help with running his (struggling) small business in a conversation with Dr. Hallowell:

GREG: It's just who I am. I'm an independent kind of guy. I've always been like this.

DR. HALLOWELL: But if I could connect you with a coach, someone who could help you with the details like scheduling and prioritizing that are causing you to fail, why not accept that help?

GREG: Because then it wouldn't be me who was succeeding. It would be me with the coach.

DR. HALLOWELL: But isn't most success like that? I couldn't have become a doctor without the help of the teachers who taught me in medical school and then the older doctors who coached me when I was a young doctor.

GREG: That's different. I should be able to run my bait and tackle shop on my own. It's not like I'm in medical school.

DR. HALLOWELL: Running a small business is every bit as complicated as medical school, if not more so. What is it about getting help that makes you so uncomfortable?

GREG: I don't know, but it does. Doc, we had this exact same discussion when you brought up the subject of trying medication. I just want to do this on my own. I want to live my life my way, on my terms.

DR. HALLOWELL: But I want to help you see how self-defeating that approach is. Especially in today's world. *No one* is independent. *No one* is self-sufficient. We *all* depend on one another. The realistic goal in life is not to be independent, but to be *effectively interdependent.* In other words, you have to be able to give as well as get. That's how successful people operate. Why waste your time doing what you're bad at? Hire someone else to do that so you can do what you're good at.

GREG: That just goes totally against my grain.

DR. HALLOWELL: Well, that grain is going to defeat you. That grain is going to keep you from becoming the big success you could become. You have the talent to become a major player in the fishing industry; lots of people who know the business have told you that. You have the entrepreneur's edge. So use it! Don't let this refusal to accept help keep you from the success you could have.

Both of us have had this conversation with patients countless times. In our experience, the refusal to accept help is the single biggest reason for a person not to progress once an ADHD diagnosis has been made. That's why it's so important to find the right difficult. As Jon and Greg and too many others' experience shows, if it is the wrong difficult, we can spend years, even decades, in frustrating and foolish pursuit of the impossible. (The same principle holds for marriage and other relationships, by the way.)

Once you have assessed your strengths—either through our ten-question assessment or through the Kolbe Index—you should have a better idea of the overlap between what you're good at and what you love to do. Neither of us can coach you on doing your own right kind of difficult—that's your own unique genius at work. But we *can* coach you on how to make your environment fertile soil for growing that talent once you identify it. That's the subject of the next chapter.

* These tests, which require a fee, can be found at Kolbe.com/TakeA and Kolbe.com/TakeY. A more specific Kolbe test is Kolbe's OPgig career program (OPgig.com), which can help pinpoint the right fit for your career.

CHAPTER 6

Create Stellar Environments

From the moment the idea of what we now call ADHD came into being, people wondered how much of it was caused by the environment and how much changing the environment might help the problems that come with it. Dr. Charles Bradley himself, the doctor who first gave a medication, amphetamine, to children to treat what we now call ADHD in 1937, ran his ward on principles of environmental engineering. In addition to medication, he tried regulating the lighting and experimenting with the staff's clothing—all to see what various changes in their environment might do for his patients.

Now that we've expanded ADHD to include VAST characteristics, and since, strictly speaking, medication is only for people who have diagnosed ADHD, the following questions become all the more relevant: What constitutes the best environment, or what we call a stellar environment, for a person who has attention issues? And how much difference does creating such an environment make?

THE IMPACT OF ENVIRONMENT

The short answer: Environment matters a great deal. All kinds of research now makes clear that our environment—including our diet, exposure to toxins, chronic stress, and many other factors—can change the way our genes get "expressed." In lay terms, that means how you live is a determinant of whether or not you get a disease to which you are genetically predisposed. In other words, your environment is a powerful tonic—for better and for worse.

Many adults never discover they have ADHD until their environment dramatically changes. For example, when a woman gives birth to or adopts her first child, the demands on her organizational skills coupled with a loss of sleep (and, if she's given birth, bodily changes) really upset the applecart of her environment. Without the calm and order of her pre-baby life, she feels frenzied and unproductive. Often Mom will be able to right the cart or find new ways of instilling order and calm into her day. Eventually—and especially when she gets some help and some good sleep—her productivity and equanimity return. But sometimes what the world sees as garden-variety new motherhood or "mommy brain" points to underlying ADHD, and only the upheaval of an environmental change reveals it.

Another example is the change that comes from stepping onto the next rung of school—whether in grade school or college or graduate school. Take medical school, which we know all too well. Suddenly the student, who has done so well in school that he or she got into medical school in the first place, must cope with demands upon his or her brain like never before. The new pace of learning—like trying to sip water from a firehose, it's often said—takes over everything, making it hard for the student to maintain his or her previously healthy and helpful practices, sleep, nutrition, and regular exercise among them. Maybe, like the new mother above, this student will find her footing. Maybe she will not—and soon discover underlying ADHD, get diagnosed, and get help. But this situation is a breeding ground for VAST as well—a culturally induced state of mind that once turned on is hard to turn off, especially if the environment remains unhealthy.

HOW TO ORGANIZE YOUR ENVIRONMENT

There are elements of your environment you obviously can't control. A new mother can't ever fully control when her baby sleeps and wakes or when the baby will need to be fed or held or changed. And new academic or career challenges are what they are; you have to try to keep up. But there are things in our environment that we absolutely *can* control, and if attention issues are in play, you absolutely must. In addition to connection, exercise, and stress reduction—which are so important that we cover them in other chapters (see chapters 4 and 7)—there are five areas of your environment that we would have you focus on for yourself or your child: daily structure, nutrition, sleep, populate your world with positivity, and accept and find the right help.

Daily Structure

Creating structure isn't something that usually comes naturally to someone with ADHD or characteristics of VAST. Abiding by and learning to like it, even less so. Indeed, structure is more likely something that you resist. Being free and a nonconformist is, after all, in our bones. But there is almost no more important and helpful lifestyle hack for us than engineering structure. Structure provides the walls of the bobsled run. Without it you careen off into disaster. Neglect it at your peril!

But don't be intimidated by it. Take heart in knowing that you probably already have some structure to your day in the form of daily habits: You probably brush your teeth and shower most days, we trust you say please and thank you, and with luck you put a napkin on your lap when you eat and take your plate to the dishwasher or sink when you're done. You have these good habits because someone made a point of explaining their importance. If you don't have these good habits, it's never too late to put them in place. You can effect change for yourself in many other ways, too.

Let's start with the proverbial low-hanging fruit: having a schedule and a to-do list. Creating structure with these two age-old strategies will help you plan, prioritize, be on time more often, and procrastinate less. Just the simple act of sitting down to write or type out a schedule or to-do list will help, because any and every time you itemize the tasks on your plate, you are neurologically reinforcing their importance.

If you're an adult, there is no shortage of scheduling and reminder hardware (notebooks, sticky notes, handheld tape recorders) and software (apps and alarms that notify you in advance of your having to be somewhere or complete something), so there is really no excuse not to set up your own simple (or elaborate) system. Paying attention to the notes and pings is another story. How many times have we been alerted or reminded and, because we've fully intended to follow through, turned the alarm or alert off…only to realize hours later that our mind took off on another track and we missed the proverbial (or literal) train? This happens to "neurotypicals" too, but it's an all-too-frequent hallmark of the ADHD mind for sure. The trick is to set up backup reminders and systems—even in the form of asking a partner or spouse to call or nudge you to help keep you on task.

But of course you can't set up a reminder system for *everything* you need to do—that might mean having an alarm or alert go off all day long (which is not ideal for another reason—see below on turning off electronic devices)! And it's not good for partner or spousal dynamics to ask another person to be the perpetual nag. Instead, start small: Pick one or two regularly scheduled commitments or expected tasks and set up a structure to help you follow through. Experiment with what works for you until you hit on it. With every appointment kept or chore completed, you'll get a little hit of self-satisfaction, and probably a lot of positive feedback from the people around you, too. That kind of feedback reward also reinforces your desire to get more of it and will help motivate your continued attention to that schedule and list.

If you're the parent of a child with ADHD or VAST tendencies, you'll likely want to be the keeper of these schedules and the setter of routines on your child's behalf, as well as be the alert/alarm/reminder to keep them on task. This isn't the same as helicopter parenting—you don't have to hover and fix and solve everything for your child. Instead, think of your role as like the bumpers on a pinball machine, the structure that keeps their energies and wild ideas just a little more in check. Put simply: All children do better when they know who is in charge. Knowing that they are not gives them a sense of security and order. The same goes for adults, to a certain extent—having a clear chain of command at work, for instance, is both orienting and especially helpful to the employee with ADHD.

As much as we want to drive home the importance of creating regular and clear expectations for your child's time, it's also critical that you build time for unstructured and uninhibited play into your child's daily schedule! Running around, moving, imagining, making—this is the work of childhood, and for the ADHD or VAST mind, this venting and creating time is all that much more needed.

It's hard to know when a child is old enough to take on the responsibility of structure making—the age will be different for every child. When you do cede control, do so incrementally so that you can be sure your child is ready for each new responsibility.

A note of caution: We can't deny that electronic devices can be helpful in creating and maintaining structure for adults and kids alike. But beware the rabbit hole of Internet and social media browsing! Being able to flit from one topic to the next to the next with just the touch of a key or swipe of a screen can give a jolt of stimulation (lights, colors, pictures, ideas!), which is, of course, a balm to our boredom-averse brains.

Recognizing your tendency to get sucked into the Internet vortex is the first step to controlling that impulse. But then do something about it: Adults should try to limit their screen time by turning the device off or putting it aside for several hours of every day (doing so as a family policy makes this easier), and definitely keep screens away from where you sleep. Charge your phone or tablet in another room overnight if your job doesn't require you to be "on call."

A child with ADHD or VAST tendencies should be kept from regular screen use for as long as the parents can resist their pleas for it. Because once you've caved in and given your child a screen of her own, there is very little room to turn back. As with when to give your child more responsibility for her own daily schedule, when to give a child a screen is going to be different for every family. But whenever that is, be sure to set clear boundaries around screen use, including times when it will not be available or on. And definitely, definitely confiscate the device at night (see Sleep, page 87).

And a note of encouragement: Rewards work much better for the ADHD mind than do consequences. So whether you're an adult working on structure for yourself or a parent maintaining it for a child, build little rewards into the systems you contrive. As mentioned earlier, getting praise from others is always nice (parents and teachers, take note!), but why not also give yourself or your child something of personal value when you complete a big task or consistently remember a bunch of small ones?

To help guide you toward building a structure that is ADHD- or VAST-friendly—at home, in your child's classroom, or at work—keep the following punch list of must-haves in mind:

STELLAR ENVIRONMENTS AT HOME

You have the most control over your home environment. Strive for your home to be a safe haven and happy place—for you and/or for your child. Key elements include:

- Playful attitude.
- Permission for everyone to be real and genuine.
- Enough structure, schedule, and rules to avoid confusion and chaos.
- Meals together daily, with whoever lives in the home; food can bring us together.
- Worry together; no one should ever worry alone.
- Encourage self-assertion and speaking up no matter what.
- Never go to bed angry.
- Have pets if you possibly can.
- Laughter, lots of laughter.
- But no ridicule or teasing, no matter how much fun they may be.
- Honesty, honesty, honesty. No phony baloney.
- But go easy on the brutal honesty. Keep it kind and gentle.
- Make a point of expressing gratitude; in the soil of love and gratitude, great and lasting joy takes root and grows.
- Cheer for one another.
- Add to this list what you and the troupe you live with, whoever they may be, value most.

STELLAR LEARNING ENVIRONMENTS

You may not have control over where your child goes to school—or precious little choice, anyway—but you can still advocate for the following in your child's classroom:

- Low-fear, high-trust atmosphere.
- Shaming not allowed.
- Rules of the room are clear. Even better: They are posted on the wall.
- A seating arrangement that promotes connection with others.
- The Socratic method of teaching. That is, dialogue and asking/answering questions to get to information. A top-down, I lecture/you listen structure is not compatible with the ADHD mind.
- Project-based learning as much as possible.
- Innovation and initiative encouraged.
- Frequent breaks for exercise during class, e.g., standing up, dancing, jogging in place, stretching.
- A teacher and an administration that encourage the identification of strengths.

STELLAR WORKING ENVIRONMENTS

Read this list with an eye toward where you work now. Does it make the grade? If not, it is time to begin looking for a working environment that meets your needs.

- Low-fear, high-trust, from the top on down through the ranks.
- Structured, organized, but not regimented.
- Workspace configuration that encourages connecting with others.
- Permission to be honest.
- An organizational or a corporate policy against gossip and backbiting.
- Clear lines of authority and communication.
- Clearly stated policies on a range of important topics: vacations, time off, harassment, personal email and texting.
- Low use of the human resources department and high use of working

things out with colleagues directly and privately (except if there's harassment—then HR should have your back!).

- Permission to be who you are, and the acknowledgment of both your weaknesses and your strengths.
- The capacity for everyone to take initiative, exert control over what they do, and get credit for what they do.
- Management makes an explicit effort to match workers' talents with tasks.
- Management clearly states and explains expectations.

Nutrition

How you fuel your body really matters. Give it good-quality "gas" (food), and your engine (body) will, barring disease or accident, run more smoothly. Of course, there's always conflicting advice about the best kind of diet. Whether your concern is weight loss, heart health, anti-inflammation, or animal welfare, there is a whole library's worth of books written about all kinds of diets and all kinds of "very best" combinations of nutrients.

But there should be no argument about what's the best fuel for the ADHD brain. We know a lot about what kinds of foods contribute to hyperactivity or substandard performance of your "machinery." And it's really not that complicated!

In general, it's best to stick to whole foods. Whole grains are better than processed grains; fresh foods are better than commercially preserved and packaged ones. Avoid processed foods, junk foods, any foods that contain additives, preservatives, and colorings.

The more veggies and fruits the better. Healthy oils and fats = good. Trans fats = bad. Steer clear of fruit juices, because they're mainly sugar (see below) and empty calories. Your body also needs good protein like unprocessed meats, fish, nuts, and eggs.

Drink lots of water. Or tea. We also love coffee, as caffeine is the best over-the-counter focus medication that there is. Just drink it in moderation and watch for side effects: elevated heart rate, irregular heartbeat, lots of trips to the bathroom (it's a laxative and a diuretic), insomnia, agitation, and irritability. These are all signs you've drunk too much coffee!

And then this all-important piece of advice: Avoid sugar. Sugar promotes the production and release of dopamine, and the ADHD brain loves a squirt of dopamine. Unfortunately, as good as that initial influx of dopamine might feel —you're energized, cheery, satisfied—you have to keep ingesting sugar to keep up that feeling. That's the reason for the gallon of ice cream at midnight, the jumbo Reese's Pieces in the movie theater, sauces and gravies on everything, cookies galore. Not only is this bad for your waistline, but the post-sugar/post-dopamine crash of mood and satiety feels terrible.

Aside from its low nutritional value and its being a temptation for people with ADHD, most of us who have a lot of experience agree that for some kids, sugar triggers disruptive behavior, though for other kids it's no problem. You have to be your own investigator. If your child goes to a birthday party, eats cake and ice cream and drinks Coke, and comes home like a ballistic missile, well, next time cut out the sugar or don't go to the party or...be prepared for a ballistic missile.

Some people with ADHD or symptoms of VAST do better when they eliminate dairy (lactose) or go on a gluten-free diet. The best way to find out is to try. Obviously, if you are gluten or lactose intolerant, you may already know it, but some people who are not strictly gluten or lactose intolerant, children and adults alike, do much better once they get on one of those restricted diets.

Some forty years ago, Dr. Benjamin Feingold championed an entire diet that was supposed to cure ADHD. It was a complex elimination diet that excluded sweeteners, additives, colorings, and many foods that contain salicylates, like cherries, almonds, tea, and tomatoes. Once a child gets on the diet and sees improvement, you start adding back the foods you eliminated, one at a time, so that you end up knowing which foods you can tolerate and which foods make your symptoms worse.

Like many people trying to introduce something new, Feingold took his diet too far, became too doctrinaire, and fell out of favor. But, as with many new programs, there was much merit to his plan. We've seen certain kids benefit tremendously from the Feingold diet, probably because of an underlying sensitivity or allergy to the foods that were eliminated.

There are some supplements everyone can agree to recommend: a multivitamin; vitamin D; magnesium; B complex; vitamin C (ascorbic acid, as well as Connect!); calcium; zinc.

Beyond that, there are a host of ADHD brain potions marketed by some reliable people and some shady ones. Because supplements are not regulated by the FDA, it's the Wild West out there. One authoritative book we recommend that explores a host of natural treatments is *Non-drug Treatments for ADHD,* by Richard Brown and Patricia Gerbarg. It is an outstanding book written by two top doctors who have no ax to grind or product to peddle.

There is one supplement that we recommend specifically and take ourselves: OmegaBrite.[*1] Developed more than twenty years ago by a Harvard-educated doctor named Carol Locke, OmegaBrite is an omega-3 fatty acid supplement that we feel confident is pharmaceutical-grade and free of contaminants like mercury.

The reason fatty acids are good for your brain, and hence for ADHD, is that the myelin sheaths that wrap around your neurons like rubber coating around electric wires are made of fat. Maintaining that fatty composition requires essential fatty acids. "Essential" means your body can't synthesize them; you have to ingest them. Unless you eat a ton of salmon, mackerel, anchovies, and sardines, you do not get enough essential fatty acids in your diet.

CBD

CBD—short for *cannabidiol*—is an extract from the cannabis plant. Yes, the same plant from which marijuana is made. It's quite the fad—now recommended for everything from bad breath to lumbago to prenuptial jitters —but we urge you not to dismiss it. In many ways it is the Next Big Thing in supplements.

When we were in medical school, one of the most exciting new discoveries was that of the *endogenous opiate receptor system*—the revelation that our brains had receptors for opiates built into them. Shortly thereafter came the discovery of endorphins, short for *endogenous morphine,* that is, the body's ability to produce morphine (which is what the runner's high is all about).

Some fifty years later, we now understand that the body has an *endogenous cannabinoid system* as well, which is a big deal, opening the door to a host of possible treatments for anxiety, pain, seizures, addiction, and, yes, ADHD.

For our purposes, the main application of cannabinoids so far appears to be in treating the anxiety that so often accompanies both ADHD and VAST. Perhaps by interacting with the *gabaminergic system,* CBD can relieve anxiety. Don't be put off by the big word. GABA is just a molecule, a neurotransmitter that drugs like the benzodiazepines (Valium, Xanax, Klonopin, and others) and alcohol promote. In the right doses it can be calming.

OmegaBrite also manufactures a CBD product called OmegaBrite CBD, which they began selling in March 2020. Early reports are that it is calming without being sedating. Dr. Hallowell takes it every day and reports that it reduces his reactivity, his tendency to get annoyed too quickly.

Sleep

Has it really come to the point where we have to urge people to sleep? It used to be that people had to be urged to wake up; now we have to urge people to go to bed. Especially us stimulation seekers who have ADHD or VAST. We don't like to leave the party, or to turn off our devices, and so we stay up way too late. But your brain will not function at 100 percent—or even close to it—if you do not get enough sleep.

How much sleep is enough? The amount of sleep it takes for you to wake up without an alarm clock. That's your physiological requirement for sleep. Try to get that much and your brain will repay you; your body will as well. Insufficient sleep is associated with increased risk of obesity, depression, high blood pressure, depressed immune function (which can lead to cancer), and anxiety disorders.

A specific sleep disorder called *sleep apnea* can actually cause a syndrome that looks just like ADHD. Sleep apnea is in what's called the "differential diagnosis" of ADHD, the list of conditions that can mimic ADHD. Also on that list are hyper- and hypothyroidism; depression; caffeinism (drinking too much coffee or other caffeinated beverages); bipolar disorder; anxiety disorders; pheochromocytoma (tumor of the adrenal gland that causes it to secrete large amounts of adrenaline); substance use disorders; post-traumatic stress disorder; and the carrying of too many secrets and too much shame (not a formal diagnosis, but we see it a lot). All of these conditions can not only mimic ADHD but also accompany it.

If a person has sleep apnea, getting it treated can basically cure what had looked like ADHD. You get this diagnosis by going to a sleep lab, which can be found in most hospitals. You suspect the diagnosis if you typically wake up still tired, if you are overweight (although thin people can have sleep apnea too), and if you are particularly prone to irritability.

While medications can help a person get to sleep, there is a relatively new device that is FDA-approved for insomnia, as well as depression and anxiety. We have also found it helpful in some patients—of all ages—with ADHD. It is called the Fisher Wallace Stimulator. It causes no side effects of note, nor is it in any way habit-forming. The device uses a mild form of alternating current to stimulate key neurotransmitters, including serotonin, dopamine, and beta-endorphin, and lower cortisol, the stress hormone. It is safe and easy to use by patients of all ages and is available upon the recommendation of anyone licensed for healthcare in the state in which they practice. Dr. Hallowell has prescribed it to several dozen patients. While not all of them have found benefit, most have, not only for the approved conditions but for ADHD as well. And since anxiety and depression, as well as insomnia, are common conditions that coexist with ADHD, the stimulator is an excellent non-medication alternative to consider. Go to Fisherwallace.com for testimonials as well as references.[2]

HOW TO PRACTICE SLEEP HYGIENE

Sleep labs can prove the efficacy of these recommendations; your own experience no doubt backs them up. You'll sleep longer and better if you:

- Turn off electronics at least one hour before you hit the hay to give your brain the needed time to slow down and become less stimulated.
- Charge electronic devices overnight outside your bedroom.
- Make your bedroom as dark as possible. The absence of light is the key

signal to your circadian rhythm that it's time to wind down.

- Turn down the heat. Or open a window a bit to get some fresh, cool air, or turn on a fan or an air conditioner.

Populate Your World with Positivity

So far we've been talking about things you can largely control—the structure of your day, what goes into your mouth, when you put your head on a pillow. But other people are part of your environment too, and you can only minimally control their actions or outlooks. But you can choose who you'll allow into your world and, to a degree, who you will spend time with. So choose wisely.

For a child, if you have the luxury of options, this means choosing a school that believes in helping him or her work from strengths. See page 68 for our recommended brief strengths assessment and share your child's answers with the school. Make sure that strengths assessment is part of your child's "record" so that everyone who comes into contact with him or her has that baseline understanding. Even if you don't have a choice of schools—whether because of finances or geography—sharing the list of your child's strengths is a gentle way to advocate for his or her needs and can initiate a positive conversation with a school or teacher who has yet to appreciate what's going on.

There are other things to look for in a school, or to ask of a school you're stuck with. Our punch list can be found in the Daily Structure discussion on page 78. One thing to reiterate: Impress upon the school administration and staff your child's need for stimulation—so they can provide opportunities to get up and move around and can try to tailor some of their teaching to your child's expressed interests.

For an adult, your workplace might surround you with positive, understanding, appreciative-of-your-talents types. If so, wonderful! But if the list (again, in Daily Structure, page 78) of circumstances that make for a stellar working environment doesn't match your daily experience, you'd do yourself a favor by keeping an eye out for a job that's a better fit.

We realize that's a tall order—especially in a down economy (as at this writing). So what else can you do to be sure you populate your environment with positivity? Choose your friends and partner with great care!

We don't have statistics to back this up, but our anecdotal evidence is overwhelming: People with ADHD and VAST often make the mistake of falling for train wrecks. That's because helping and saving people in distress is highly stimulating. Our advice: Try to fall for a stable person who is also stimulating. They really do exist.

More generally, steer clear of people who bring you down, who gossip, who are predominantly cynical and negative. That's not to say you have to associate only with cheerful optimists. Some of our best friends are dyed-in-the-wool curmudgeonly pessimists, but they exude warmth nonetheless. What you want to avoid is people who drain you of all your positive energy. Notice how you feel when you leave a person. That's a good indicator of whether it's worth spending more time with that person.

Accept and Find the Right Help

The idea of asking for and finding the right kind of help is a cousin to one of our overarching rules: Never worry alone. When the demands upon you exceed your ability to meet them, get help in the right places from the right people.

Most people understand that asking for help is not a sign of weakness, at least in most contexts. If you're a new parent, for instance, there's usually no shame in asking for advice or help from your parents or friends, or from your new baby's pediatrician. There is certainly still stigma around seeking help for postpartum depression, but even that is dissipating as more and more women raise their hands to say they've experienced it and more and more doctors screen for signs of it. So it should be for asking for help for ADHD or VAST. As we say all the time to our patients: Don't just tough it out. Work smart, not just hard.

The social limitations of ADHD/VAST can be painful and disabling, so it is important to take this step seriously.

SOCIAL COACHING

While doing your best to associate with stellar people makes a lot of sense, you can't completely control the people you must associate with. Whether you are a child in school, thrown in with a random new group every year, or an adult in the workplace, being asked to collaborate with some people you don't much like, knowing how to get along with anyone who comes your way leads to a happier and more successful life.

This is where new research comes to the rescue. Not so long ago we did not have reliable methods of teaching children (let alone adults) how to get along with others, but now we do.

Starting with Pavlov and his famous dogs in Russia, then coming to America with B. F. Skinner and his equally famous rats at Harvard, the *behaviorist* movement liberated us from the notion that free will alone determines human actions. According to the behaviorists, if a person is intrusive, or silly, or rude, that does not mean they *intend* to be that way, nor, more important, that they are destined to continue to be that way.

The research into behaviorism spawned an entire arm of treatment that is still widely and successfully used today: *applied behavioral analysis* (ABA). Often used to treat autism, ABA can also be used to change habits of any kind, learn new habits, develop new routines, toilet-train toddlers, even manage large organizations. The mission of ABA is to develop a set of skills that will help an individual do better in life.

But another approach can be more effective in teaching us how to read a social scene rather than just change habits and behaviors. This method helps people *understand* their behavior rather than just change it and is therefore aptly called *social learning*. Instead of just focusing on skills, the practitioner tries to help a child understand what's going on in a social situation and learn accordingly.

If you have a child who just can't figure out how to get along, who doesn't "get" being in a group in the way that some other child doesn't "get" word problems in math, then you need a specialist who can go beyond ABA training skills, who can do more than tell the child what actions to ape, what words to recite, what motions to go through. You need a coach who can help your child think and feel through all the various steps that combine to create the amazingly complex interaction called "getting along." This comes naturally to some children, just as skating backward does to some. But to others it is utterly foreign, just as some children fall on their butts when they try to skate backward. However, there is a knack to both that can be broken down into learnable steps. *You do not have to be born with the knack. You can learn it inductively, rather than memorize it or have it conditioned into you.* This is the great discovery that separates social learning from behaviorist training.

The two groups, the ABA people and the social learning folks, argue over who is right, which is counterproductive. Each group has a great deal to offer. If you want to quit smoking or overeating or to break some other habit, go to an ABA specialist. But if you want to learn how to get along with others, seek out a social learning specialist, sometimes also called a social learning coach. One truly excellent coach, Caroline Maguire, wrote an excellent book that we urge you to consult: *Why Will No One Play with Me? The Play Better Plan to Help Children of all Ages Make Friends and Thrive.*

It's worth noting that changing behavior through ABA is often more than enough. But sometimes you want to go deeper, to help a child—or anyone else—understand cognitively and emotionally where they are and who they are in social situations, recognize their options, and decide for themselves what they want to do. Once they learn how to decide for themselves what they want to do, rather than put on reflexive behaviors they've been conditioned to show, real growth ensues. ABA is surface; social learning is deep. ABA is more or less robotic; social learning helps you understand social situations and respond according to your own desires and values. ABA is more mechanical; social learning is more supple and human. By coaching children in how to understand social situations and how to develop different ways of handling them, you can teach them not only how to do it but also enjoy doing so that the interaction is not just a matter of going through the motions.

---

*1 OmegaBrite has sponsored Dr. Hallowell's podcast *Distraction*.

*2 Neither Dr. Hallowell nor Dr. Ratey receives any compensation from Fisher Wallace.

CHAPTER 7

Move to Focus, Move to Motivate: The Power of Exercise

Have a big paper due or presentation to give? Need to study for an important test? Here's a pro tip: Take a run around the block, go up and down the stairs in your house, just do something to get yourself moving. You'll definitely notice the difference in your ability to focus and settle into the needed zone. Better yet, make it a regular habit and consider it a necessary dose of medicine to keep you functioning as your best self.

For getting and staying on track, exercise is one of the most powerful non-medical tools we have and an important first line of defense. Beyond making your cardiologist happy, or looking better in a bathing suit, one of the most fascinating and beneficial effects of exercise is that it prepares the brain to expand, learn, and change better than any other human activity. It improves mood and motivation, reduces anxiety, regulates emotions, and maintains focus.

From depression to anxiety as well as for ADHD and VAST symptoms, exercise is just what the doctor should order.

SEEING IS BELIEVING

In the very early 1980s, a patient we'll call David came to see Dr. Ratey.

A professor at an elite New England university, David had been incredibly productive and successful at work—he'd written many books and published dozens of papers, and he was a frequent keynote speaker around the world. He'd also been a runner all his life; the marathon was his preferred distance. Some months prior to coming to Dr. Ratey, however, David had twisted his knee and was forced to stop training and competing. His pace was now slowed to a walk, which he did gingerly at that.

David had recently emerged from a brief depression related to his injury, which was understandable, since he was forced to step away from his lifelong habit and passion in order to heal, but he was more concerned with other challenges he was now facing. David couldn't focus on his work, and his personal life was a mess. This formerly high-functioning, multitasking professor was procrastinating at every turn, didn't return phone calls, was getting unduly angry with his longtime girlfriend for stupid reasons, wasn't seeing friends, and his work on his many projects was grinding to a halt. He could not get started on, nor stay with, his writing and reading, was forgetting appointments, and was uncharacteristically disorganized. It seemed that the change in his routine and environment had revealed his underlying ADHD. Running had been a lifelong coping mechanism.

Because David was eager to reverse his downward spiral—desperate, really, to be more like his old self—and because he could not yet get back to running as a salve, Dr. Ratey prescribed Ritalin. It had an immediate positive effect. Within six months, David's ability to start and finish work had returned and he was much better able to modulate his emotions, which was helping matters in the relationship department.

When David's knee healed and he was finally able to get back into his running routine, he and Dr. Ratey agreed that the time was right to taper off the Ritalin, which he did without any disruption to his work drive. In the coming years, David occasionally used a small dose of Ritalin to sharpen his focus, but his return to running was his own kind of medication, a truly effective treatment for his previously unrecognized ADHD.

THE SCIENCE

So what exactly is going on when you lace up your sneakers and go for a jog, or hit the gym, or turn up the music to dance?

The benefits of getting your heart rate up are many, and perhaps one of the most important is the release of a protein called *brain-derived neurotropic factor,* or BDNF. We think of this as Miracle-Gro for the brain, as it creates a fertile environment to grow new neurons, connectors, and positive pathways. Additionally, when we exercise, we are using more nerve cells than in any other human activity. The more we move, the more those cells are clicking away and firing. When they fire, they release more neurotransmitters to carry information from one nerve cell to the next, creating a boost in dopamine and norepinephrine, which play a major role in regulating our attention system.

In fact, the role of the stimulants and antidepressants we prescribe for ADHD is to increase the concentration of dopamine and norepinephrine in the brain, as they contribute to maintaining alertness and increasing and sustaining focus and motivation. One of the ongoing findings in ADHD research is that some of the gene differences associated with ADHD are related to faulty dopamine and norepinephrine machinery, so a blast of exercise is like taking a stimulant that corrects this deficit for the moment. We see an aroused and attentive being.

When you exercise, the clunky connectomes in the default mode network become smoother, allowing for easier and more complete transitions into the task-positive network, where we access our frontal cortex. Remember, the frontal cortex is the CEO of the brain. When you get yourself moving, this area is "sparked," turning your attention system on and allowing you to stay focused and on task.

The best part? You don't have to be a marathon runner like David to get the benefits. In 2018, a paper out of Spain looked at a range of studies over twelve years using exercise as an intervention to treat ADHD. The team looked at more than seven hundred individuals from eight countries. After doing just twenty to thirty minutes of moderately paced exercise, those subjects experienced an increased reaction speed and precision of response, helping them to "switch gears" to focus with greater strength and accuracy.

Additionally, 65 percent of the people significantly improved their planning and organization skills; this, after just a single episode of exercising for twenty to thirty minutes.

SUCCESS IN THE CLASSROOM

Some of the most creative and outside-the-box thinking about using exercise to help those with ADHD is coming from our schools and educators. Teachers will be the first to tell you that almost no child can sit still for hours upon hours, nor can most adults for that matter. It becomes even more apparent when you have an increasing number of pupils in the classroom who are ADHD or struggling with learning problems.

In Saskatoon, Canada, eighth-grade teacher Allison Cameron faced an even greater challenge. She worked at City Park Collegiate, a school known as a place of last resort. This is where kids who don't fit in at other schools in the district are sent to get back on track. Many live in poverty with little support, were born with fetal alcohol syndrome or have gotten into drugs and alcohol themselves, or have taken a wrong turn in a multitude of both academic and personal ways. It was here she was tasked with heading up a behavior management program with the toughest of even these tough students. As Allison tells it, "They were red-flagged as the worst-behaved students in the division. In order to be red-flagged for the program, students had to have a rap sheet pages long for fighting, defiance, disrespect."

But that wasn't all this young, energetic teacher was dealing with. The majority of her students were reading and writing at least four grade levels below where they should have been, and close to 100 percent had been diagnosed with ADHD and were on medication for it. Absenteeism was rampant, and with the majority of her kids battling major attention problems, getting them to sit still long enough to learn was nearly impossible.

Allison had seen with previous students the power of exercise to help with both behavior and cognition. She decided to give it a shot with her new charges. "On the first day of school, I suggested we go for a run to see if we could work on some of their irrational and combative behaviors....They refused to run, so I settled with taking them for a walk. A thirty-minute walk turned into a two-hour stroll for some and a free pass for two others to go get high. After that day, I realized I had no choice but to keep them inside the school to get their heart rates up."

Undeterred, Allison persuaded a gym owner she knew to assist in getting some key pieces of equipment donated to her cause. Soon her classroom was crowded: she had eight treadmills and six stationary bikes, and also fourteen heart rate monitors. That's when things started to change. "I could see the potential of the students and I knew if I could just get their heart rates up for more than ninety seconds, we would all be much happier."

Allison says that using the equipment herself was an important first step in getting reluctant students to buy into the program. Also, their choice was between getting on a treadmill or bike and sitting in a chair and doing math, so it was no wonder they strapped on their donated heart rate monitors. "I explained that all I was requiring them to do was elevate their heart rates to sixty-five to seventy-five percent of their maximum. It was a novel concept for the students and they started to see it as fun."

During her forty-five-minute classes, Allison got her students up and running for twenty minutes and then got down to classwork, which was actually a net gain of learning time, since she had been previously spending the first thirty minutes of class dealing with discipline problems. Now the kids were up and moving, regulating their emotions while turning on their attention systems. When they got off the equipment, they could sit still, absorb information, and actually learn something in addition to feeling better about themselves. "They were quitting smoking, losing weight, many were able to reduce or get off of their medication, and students were telling me how much better they felt. They were coming to school every day so they could go on a treadmill!"

Attendance increased, and in the second semester, suspensions dropped to zero. To top it off, test scores skyrocketed. "On average, their reading levels, sight words, and comprehension had grown four full grade levels in four months!" says Allison with pride. "These students became the biggest advocates for the program, bragging to their peers and family about their successes."

While it's impossible for every classroom to have treadmills and bikes, the news of this kind of success is spreading, and many schools and teachers recognize the benefits of "brain breaks," or allowing kids to get up from their desks and do some jumping around. Also, many school administrators recognize the importance of good old-fashioned recess and are protecting that free time—on the grounds that it improves learning and behavior—from those who would do away with it in the name of more class time.

TIME-IN—A NEW KIND OF TIME-OUT

Another innovation increasingly used in classrooms is a spin on a traditional "time-out." A "time-out" asks a student to sit in a study hall or quietly outside the principal's office (or, in your house, in their room), but a "time-in" engages them in some sort of physical activity. A time-in can be as simple as getting a child on a stationary bike to restore emotional regulation, but some elementary schools send kids to hop on an Urban Rebounder or mini trampoline until they have calmed down. Others have the child walk up and down stairs, or simply send the child on an errand to deliver something to another part of the building.

One Boston school connected to the juvenile justice system, where most of the kids have ADHD, has really taken the message to heart. Inspired by Dr. Ratey's 2008 book *Spark: The Revolutionary New Science of Exercise and the Brain,* they've established a "Ratey Room," which has a *Dance Dance Revolution* setup, an Urban Rebounder, and some additional exercise equipment. When students act up, they are sent to the Ratey Room. As they sweat, they are getting their emotions in check and their brains turned on, putting themselves back on track and ready to learn. You might think that kids would be purposely disruptive in order to get sent to this fun-sounding space, but in reality these kids—like all kids—want to stay in the regular classroom with their peers. Being sent to the Ratey Room isn't something they gun for, but it is something from which they greatly benefit.

This kind of innovation is happening on the other side of the globe as well. Tatsuo Okada, a Ph.D. from UCLA, is at the forefront of using exercise and play to help those in Japan with ADHD, autism, and other brain differences.

Because physical activity had helped him with his own ADHD, and because he was familiar with and inspired by Dr. Ratey's *Spark,* Okada started an after-school "Spark Center" in Tokyo in 2013 to get kids moving. Buoyed by grateful parents, and the Japanese government's acknowledgment of the positive results, Okada has now opened eighteen locations around Japan and has still more plans to expand.

Visit one of these brightly lit centers and you'll see kids running around, laughing and squealing. At first glance, it seems like a complete free-for-all. But look closer and you will see highly engaged adult trainers playfully chasing after the kids, encouraging them to do different obstacle courses or to complete a series of tasks for which they have no choice but to stay focused. The kids are actively using their attention systems, which are being further strengthened by getting their heart rates up. "The program becomes much more effective when it stimulates the child's interest and curiosity," Okada explains. "We make sure to get the child's attention, grow that interest, and move with purpose….It is interesting to observe that when a child is focused on exercise and play, his or her sensory and emotional issues almost disappear."

Any of these get-up-and-move strategies can be replicated at home, of course. Rather than punishing your child with a time-out in their room or forcing them to sit quietly, send them up and down the stairs, around the block, down to the basement to get on a mini trampoline, or turn up the music and get them dancing. One game that Okada uses can be easily replicated at home: Tape random numbers on the walls around a room, or outside on trees. Call out numbers and require kids to see how quickly they can tag them. This gets their heart rates up, which in turn lights up the task-positive network (TPN), serving to strengthen the connections between the default mode network (DMN) and TPN in the process.

A QUESTION OF BALANCE

As Dr. Hallowell's experience with Samuel (see chapter 3) illustrates, balance and coordination training can be transformative for kids with ADHD. His prescription of having the preteen do a variety of challenges, like standing on one foot with his eyes closed, balancing on a wobble board, and juggling, may have seemed strange when you first read about it, but there is hard science behind strengthening the balance and coordination of those with attention issues. And it's never too early to start. One recent study looked at two groups of high-risk preschoolers (based on their high level of ADHD symptoms) and gave one group learned balance training. Although it was a small sampling (fifteen kids in all), there was a significant improvement in attention and self-control in those who did targeted balance training compared to those who didn't.

One fitness practice that does an excellent job of incorporating balance and coordination, along with focus and discipline, is martial arts. At a 1990 conference for the faculty of schools dealing with the toughest kids in the United States, Dr. Ratey met teachers and counselors from educational facilities that today are often called wilderness programs, places where children with conduct disorders and extreme oppositional behavior are sent to "straighten out." To his surprise (remember, this was 1990), he learned that many of these programs highlighted tae kwon do or karate as a required daily course. From a distance, it might seem very risky to give kids with severe behavior problems lessons in movement that can seriously injure others. However, the counselors explained that they had very strict protocols and excellent masters who demanded that the kids execute their punches, kicks, and knee strikes with precision before moving up to the next skill level. This workout required the kids to focus, control their own bodies, and master their emotions. Combined with the physicality of martial arts, the workouts seemed to strengthen the kids' neural networks as well. The result was a drop in their disruptive and dangerous behaviors, an improvement in grades, and an all-around increase in well-being. This early result matches what we now see in other studies of adding martial arts training to ADHD treatment: real and sustained improvement in both children and adults. Finding the right instructor is important, of course, but fortunately, recognizing how much martial arts can benefit those with ADHD has not been lost on those who teach and own facilities. There are many who specialize in working with kids who have attention challenges.

YOGA AND MEDITATION

As anyone who has ever even dabbled in a yoga practice knows, with every tree pose and warrior pose, you are strengthening your balance, along with your focus. Yoga demands noticing the body and breath and making small and specific adjustments to properly align with postures. Depending on the kind of yoga you're doing, you can also get your heart rate up, which increases the benefit to your focus and learning capability.

A recent study from Taiwan looked at the effects of yoga on forty-nine ten-year-olds. Roughly half of these kids did yoga twice a week for eight weeks, and the other half—the control group—did not. The groups were given two specific attention tests both before and after the eight-week period. One of the tests is called the Determination Test, which assesses a person's reaction speed, attention deficits, and reactive stress tolerance in the presence of continuous but rapidly changing acoustic and optical stimuli. The other test, the Visual Pursuit Test, measures perception and selective attention through line-tracking challenges. In both tests, significant improvements in accuracy rate and reaction time were observed only for the group of kids who had done yoga.

While obviously less aerobically challenging than yoga, meditation has shown powerful results, and it is particularly helpful when wrestling with the pesky default mode network of our brains. Remember, this is the area where we can slip into endless destructive rumination, or find our minds wandering and pinging from thought to thought, which is often colorfully referred to in the meditation community as "monkey mind." A recent study from Yale University found that mindfulness meditation tangibly decreases activity in the DMN, dialing it down when it seems to have a destructive hold.

With regular practice, you can actually change the structure of your brain through meditation. A 2011 Harvard study found that just eight weeks of mindfulness-based stress reduction work increased the cortical thickness in the hippocampus. This is a key area of the brain that oversees our learning, memory, and emotional regulation, all important areas to strengthen for those of us with the variable attention stimulus trait.

An important part of meditation is a focus on breath. Becoming aware of your breathing, through breath counting and other techniques, requires targeted attention, which will naturally strengthen those connections to your task-positive network. As your mind starts to wander, the goal is to go back to focusing on your breathing over and over until your mind begins to become more still. There are many apps that can help you do this, including Headspace, Calm, and Mindfulness.

We also recommend what's known as the "Ha" breathing technique. It's simple but takes some focus and concentration. To begin, inhale through your nose to a count of three or four. Next, exhale through your mouth to a count of six or eight making a soft *haaaa* sound as you do so. The inhale/exhale relationship is always at a 1:2 ratio. Using this kind of forced breath technique as you settle into meditation can interrupt those unwanted ruminations, immediately turning up alertness and attention.

MOTIVATION

Some people lay out their workout clothes every night as a way to motivate themselves to exercise in the morning. Others promise themselves a reward— a kind of carrot to keep them working toward their workout goal. But there is another now proven way to motivate yourself to stick with your exercise: Imagine or recall how good it feels after you're finished.

A recent study led by Dr. Michelle Segar at the University of Michigan showed that for adults, the best long-term (defined as more than one year) motivator for exercising was stress reduction and a feeling of well-being. In other words, it's not an external goal like wanting to lose weight for your upcoming reunion or buying the gizmo you've had your eye on that really works. Instead, it's asking yourself to remember how good exercise makes you feel that keeps you moving.

One of our favorite stories at the intersection of exercise, focus, and motivation comes from a girl we'll call Lucy. Lucy was smart as a whip, but her ADHD made math difficult for her. She'd get easily frustrated—fractions, decimals, and multiplication just didn't come as easily to her as her other subjects. She didn't have the patience to sit down and tackle the problems and couldn't wrap her brain around them. This caused her to have frequent tantrums when she began her math homework.

Dr. Ratey suggested Lucy try jumping rope vigorously for five minutes before starting on her math. It clicked! Feeling less anxious, and with her brain turned on, she no longer felt as daunted by the math problems. Years later, buoyed by her success, Lucy kept at this practice in both college and nursing school. When she felt overwhelmed or frustrated with organic chemistry, physics, or an anatomy lab, she'd jump rope, which had become her "conditioned motivator." She knew that doing so would instantly reduce her stress, make her feel better, and get her brain back on track.

GET MOVING

There is no one perfect formula for the right amount of exercise or the best target heart rate to help with ADHD and VAST issues; there are too many variables. That said, we recommend that you do some sort of physical activity for at least twenty minutes every day. Make it fun and interesting, and something you will want to do again. And over the course of the week, vary what you do; different activities stimulate different parts of the brain. Of course, for those of us with ADHD, novelty is important for other reasons, since boredom is our archenemy. It's good to do a mix-and-match from the following list:

- Aerobic activity, getting your heart rate up to 70 percent max for at least twenty minutes.
- Balance training, to strengthen your cerebellum as well as your core. Yoga or using a BOSU ball are both good options.
- Focused fitness, which keeps you on point while getting your heart rate up. Zumba or other dance programs, racket or team sports, and martial arts all fit the bill.
- For overall health and fitness, strength training is also excellent, and it will naturally be incorporated into some of these activities.

- If you want extra credit, take some of your fitness choices outside in nature whenever possible.

For any and all of these exercise categories, it's always helpful to be accountable to someone, or to have a regular routine that involves someone else. Walking after dinner with your spouse, a friend, or your child who is struggling with symptoms has the added bonus of bonding time. And of course getting fit with a friend, or friends, adds an extra layer of fun.

CHAPTER 8

I

Medication: The Most Powerful Tool Everyone Fears

The number one question we hear from patients—or their parents—is "Do you believe in Ritalin?" We understand that people are really asking if we are of the school of doctors who prescribe medication to treat ADHD, but we are often tempted to be literal and reply: "Ritalin is not a religious principle!" Nor, as many would have you believe, is it an agent of the devil, aka Big Pharma.[*] Unfortunately, from Adderall to Zenzedi, the medications prescribed for ADHD have entered the realm of hot-button issues, and in that realm reason disappears. We try to bring reason back into the conversation.

A VALUABLE TOOL

Over the long haul, skill building; finding the right school or job; finding the right teacher, mentor, or mate; and developing what we call a life rife with positive connections to people, activities, and purpose matter the most, but in the short term nothing gives you the bang for your buck that medication can.

Indeed, as long as medications are prescribed and taken properly, they afford by far the most immediate (in some cases within an hour of taking them) and effective benefit of any treatment there is; they are a hugely valuable tool in our therapeutic toolbox.

Whether to prescribe a medication (on the doctor's part) and whether to take one (on the patient's part) ought to be based on empirical studies, not on faith or the Internet or a gut feeling. Sure, base the decision on what you hope for, but also on clear evidence you can see. To that end, when one of us prescribes a medication to help a patient with ADHD, we do so as an act of science, a decision rooted in our reading of carefully conducted randomized controlled trials and with confidence that the efficacy of the medication is not in doubt. In 2018, a large study of studies, compiled by Dr. Samuele Cortese from the University of Southampton in the UK, looked at 133 randomized research papers on the effects of medication on ADHD. The results were conclusive that medication for ADHD is effective, not 100 percent of the time, of course (no medication works 100 percent of the time), but on average from 70 to 80 percent of the time.

People who disparage the use of medication or slander those of us who prescribe it have probably never heard the stories of abject human suffering in people of all ages that we hear every day, either in person or from people writing to us from around the world. Nor have they heard a mother or a newly treated adult cry over the amazing benefits the medication has led to in just a matter of days, ending years of needless suffering. To deplore the use of a tool that can not only relieve suffering but actually turn it into success, health, and joy, well, that's just plain ignorant, as well as cruel to the people whom it scares away from ever trying medication.

Surprisingly, many who warn against ADHD medications—or who are afraid to start one—might be unknowingly self-medicating through a stimulant like caffeine—in their daily coffee order, or in any of the energy drinks on the market (Red Bull, 5-hour Energy, Monster Energy drinks, and others). Many other softly packaged over-the-counter "drugs" (Adrafinil and ginkgo biloba supplements are popular "study drugs") are used by teens and adults to boost mood, arousal, and cognition. Unlike doctor-prescribed stimulants, these over-the-counter products are not controlled and can have various side effects, and any positive effects are often unsustainable.

ASSESSING WHEN THE TIME IS RIGHT

Even with assurances that it is powerful and safe, whether to put a child on a medication, or to go on one yourself, is a big, often agonizing decision that impacts the entire family. Which leads to another common question: "Could we try a non-pharmaceutical treatment first and then try medication if the other doesn't work?" In other words, *when* is the right time to try medication?

As you saw from our coverage of cerebellar stimulation techniques in chapter 3, we certainly do recognize the distinct merit of non-pharmaceutical treatment, even if the results will not be as immediately seen or felt. But from a strictly pharmacological standpoint, this strategy is sort of like saying "Let's try a year of squinting before we try eyeglasses."

That said, we also feel strongly that no one should take a medication, or ask their child to, unless they want to take it. Indeed, any medication works better if you *want to take it.* This is because of the placebo effect, a proven phenomenon that draws upon your mind's ability to enhance the efficacy of *any* intervention, from medication to surgery to acupuncture to exercise to contact lenses to the next meal you eat.

Before you dismiss the placebo effect—or dismiss how you should factor it into your decision about whether to take a medication for ADHD—consider how much better you do on a job you want, or even at a job interview for a job you want; consider how much better care you take of something—a dog, a car, a boat, a house—if you really wanted it; consider how much more you like your meal if you have been looking forward to trying the restaurant in which it is served, or how much more you like the movie if you picked it out, or how much more you like the president if you voted for him or her, or your boss if he or she hired you (or your employee if you did the hiring!).

Not to belabor the obvious, but this is a point most people overlook. It's really a fundamental principle of a happy and successful life. We do better when we are involved with activities and people we want to be involved with. We do worse, far worse, when forced or coerced. Like doing the right thing for the wrong reason, even the best medication will not work as well as it could if you do not want to take it. So wait as long as it takes for you or your child not only to get comfortable but to want to take medication before you start it.

THINK IN TERMS OF RISK VS. BENEFIT

A man we'll call Dan approached Dr. Ratey after a speech on ADHD he gave in California. Dan explained that his nine-year-old grandson, Steven, had just been diagnosed as having ADHD. Steven was having frequent outbursts at home; he couldn't seem to settle down at the dinner table or focus on his homework at night. He was failing in school, had already been held back a year, and was unpopular with kids in the classroom. Dan seemed confident in the clinical diagnosis, but he was also concerned that Steven's parents didn't seem to put limits on him. In addition, they were resisting Steven's doctor's recommendation to start medication. They feared that it might damage Steven in some way, in addition to further stigmatizing him, setting him apart as having a disorder. *What,* Dan asked, *should I tell them?*

A few things stood out in this all-too-common story. First, as Dr. Ratey explained to Dan, setting control and limits is essential by age nine. An adult can more easily create coping and organization mechanisms, hire a coach, and recognize the problems and talk to a therapist. A child with ADHD needs to learn boundaries with the help of a parent. Dr. Ratey also explained that given his symptoms and behaviors, it was that much more important for Steven to get outside to play and exercise. He also explained that good habits around sleep, eating, and screen time were going to be essential for Steven.

On the all-important question of medication, Dr. Ratey suggested that Steven's parents be encouraged to do a serious risk/benefit analysis. Whether just in casual conversation or more formally by making a pro/con chart together, they needed to consider how ADHD was affecting Steven's life scholastically, socially, and emotionally. Was Steven at risk of developing a self-image as a failure? Had he already done so? Was his inability to put on the brakes impacting his socialization and efforts to make friends? Did they see other ways to reverse the downward academic trajectory Steven was on, and quickly?

When making your own risk/benefit assessment, we encourage you to answer three important questions:

1. In addition to consulting my healthcare provider, have I learned as much as I can about this disorder from reputable sources?
2. Am I doing everything I can in terms of non-medical treatments (e.g., connecting, building structure into my day, getting exercise and quality sleep, eating well, meditating, and other beneficial habits)?
3. How much is this disorder negatively impacting my life or the life of a loved one?

CONSIDERING THE OPTIONS

If the answers to these questions convince you to go the route of medication for yourself or your child, you need to understand the pharmaceutical options. When we first entered the field, the choices were limited. Now they are many: stimulants, stimulant-like drugs, and what we call outlier medications, which include long-acting versions of the others. What follows in this chapter is explanation and commentary on each of these categories.

When it comes to ADHD medication, the important thing to remember is that there is no one-size-fits-all approach. The advice of Paul Wender—who was a professor at the University of Utah Medical School and someone we think of as the father of biological psychiatry—is apt here: "Some drugs work in some people, at some dose, some of the time."

The key is to be patient with your healthcare provider until you come up with a formula that works. This might entail multiple tries with multiple drugs, and as we do with our patients, combining different drugs at different times. Keep close tabs on any side effects, duration and peak of efficacy, and any shifts in impact, both positive and negative. The more your doctor knows, the easier it is to tailor an effective treatment plan.

STIMULANTS

Stimulants are the ADHD drug of choice. They have been shown to be the most effective with the fewest side effects; the 70 to 80 percent efficacy rate mentioned above is attributable mostly to the use and study of this category of medications. As with many prescription medications, there is some concern—some of it valid—about becoming addicted to stimulants and/or abusing them, though the issue is rather rare. We will get into these concerns briefly below.

Stimulants can be divided into two main categories: *methylphenidate type,* commonly packaged as Concerta, Ritalin, Focalin, Metadate, Quillivant, and OROS-MPH), and *amphetamine type,* which you might recognize as Adderall, Dexedrine, Evekeo, Vyvanse, and Mydayis.

It may seem counterintuitive to use something classified as a stimulant for a brain that already seems in hyperdrive, but that logic discounts the fact that stimulants actually raise the levels of dopamine and norepinephrine—two neurotransmitters that are off-kilter in the ADHD brain. You might say that stimulants stimulate the brain's brakes, thus giving you more control.

An increase in dopamine helps our nerve cells pass on information more "cleanly" from one to another. It helps to reduce the noise, quiet the chatterbox, and tune your brain to the right channel. If the signals aren't clear, it's easy to fall into confusion and anxiety.

Dopamine also increases our motivation. A 2020 study by the Brown University psychologist Andrew Westbrook and colleagues showed that kind of result, which many people report while taking a methylphenidate medication: an increase in the amount of available dopamine in a region deep in the brain involved in motivation (the *caudate nucleus*) and thus, as a practical matter measured in the study, a desire to tackle a difficult task. Those who were not taking a methylphenidate opted for an easier task.

There are non-pharmaceutical ways to increase dopamine—some healthy, like exercise and engaging your creativity and being connected to others or to a higher goal, and some counterproductive, like bingeing on carbs; using drugs like alcohol, cocaine, marijuana, and Xanax; or engaging in compulsive activities like gambling, shopping, sex, or workaholism. Failing to master the adaptive pursuit of dopamine leads to addictions of all kinds, but mastering it leads to success and joy.

By increasing norepinephrine (NEP) we increase arousal, making us more awake. This improves our ability to take in information from the environment, meaning that our senses are more attuned. We are better able to "read the room" and our audio and visual understanding is clearer.

Both dopamine and NEP stimulate our executive functioning, controlled by the prefrontal cortex (known as the CEO of the brain). This is where planning, sorting, sequencing what's important, helping with memory, and evaluating consequences are housed. The executive function helps us to put the brakes on: stopping inappropriate responses, impulsive actions, and getting lured into the next internal or external stimulation.

When it comes to the two types of stimulants, the difference is this: methylphenidate type drugs (like Ritalin) raise dopamine levels a little higher than NEP. In the amphetamine type drugs (like Adderall), it's the reverse. Amphetamine drugs have a greater effect on NEP than on dopamine, though also only by a small amount.

Researchers have also found a small divide in the efficacy of these classifications of drugs based on a person's age. For kids and teens, methylphenidates were found to be slightly more effective; when it comes to adults, amphetamines got the best results by a hair. Just about all the drugs tested were less well tolerated than placebos, but this is to be expected.

STIMULANT-LIKE DRUGS

As the name would imply, stimulant-like drugs act like stimulants in that they raise the levels of dopamine and norepinephrine, but they act on those systems in very different ways. Marketed as Wellbutrin, Strattera, and Norpramin, these drugs were developed as antidepressants but soon found their niche in the ADHD world. Longer-acting than stimulants, they can be used morning or night. With no abuse potential, they are a good option for those at risk for substance abuse. They are also an alternative to try for those who have side effects with stimulants. When they work, as they do for a certain segment of the ADHD population (which we cannot predict in advance), they can work beautifully. The downside is that, clinically, they have been shown not to be as effective as the stimulants for most people. Also, these drugs are slower-acting and may take a number of weeks to reach peak efficacy, in addition to having some common side effects like insomnia, agitation, dry mouth, nausea, headache, constipation, and, in the case of Norpramin, cardiac arrhythmias.

Another stimulant-like drug, modafinil (brand name Provigil), works by stimulating both the histamine network and dopamine, which makes us awake and attentive. Originally designed for narcolepsy, and popular with shift workers like night nurses and pilots, it also has benefits for some with ADHD. The pluses include working very smoothly for eight to twelve hours and having minimal side effects. It's not FDA-approved for ADHD use, so getting insurance approval can be tough, and some who take modafinil do experience anxiety and sleeplessness.

Originally released in 1966 as an antiviral agent, Amantadine is another stimulant-like medication worth mentioning. It was also originally used to help with Parkinson's symptoms like tremors, stiffness, and attention difficulties. Amantadine has an effect on the dopamine system; it acts weakly like a dopamine surrogate. It also stimulates another neurotransmitter that assists in increasing the actual concentration of dopamine. It has recently been used to treat attention difficulties in Alzheimer's, in head trauma, and in ADHD with some positive effect. While not yet FDA-approved for ADHD, it is being investigated with an eye toward full approval. The positives of Amantadine include a smooth effect that can last for up to twenty-four hours, with few side effects. It is not addictive and not a controlled substance, which means it can be prescribed with refills.

OUTLIERS

There are a number of drugs that don't fit neatly into the stimulant or stimulant-like category. We call these the outliers. Included in the outlier list are clonidine and its sister drug, guanfacine, which is sold and promoted in its long-acting form as Intuniv. These are both old blood pressure medicines that are extremely useful alone or in combination with stimulants. Their major effect is to calm agitation, aggression, and emotional hypersensitivity, along with assisting with focus and attention.

One of the reasons these outlier drugs are gaining in importance is because of a newly understood disorder called *rejection-sensitive dysphoria,* or RSD. This is extreme emotional pain triggered by the perception, real or imagined, that a person has been rejected, ridiculed, or criticized by important people in their life. RSD may also be triggered by a sense of falling short, such as failing to meet their own high standards or the expectations of others.

Rejection sensitivity is often a part of ADHD. As discussed in chapter 1, those with ADHD have a tendency to dwell on the "slights" of normal life and amplify their effect. Often, a person with RSD and ADHD is hypervigilant, trying at all costs to diminish these feelings. This can lead to misreading the cues of others, or withdrawing from their lives to avoid the anticipated slights. RSD can also lead to aggressive outbursts and temper tantrums as a person attempts to fight back against imagined threats.

William Dodson, a wonderful psychiatrist who is leading the way in helping us understand the prevalence of this disorder, says that just knowing there is a name for this feeling comforts patients. Whether it is isolated RSD or RSD that coexists with ADHD, it makes a difference to people to realize they are not alone. By naming it, they can actively attempt to tame it, staving off the downward spiral to despair. For those who are deeply affected by RSD, about one in three people feel relief from this despair with a combination of clonidine and guanfacine. While there is no risk of abuse with these medications, they can cause a patient's blood pressure to drop significantly. And stopping the regime should be done slowly, as otherwise it can cause a significant rise in blood pressure and pulse.

It's been more than four decades since we entered the field, and while there haven't been many seismic shifts in ADHD medication in the ensuing years, one game changer has been the concept of "long-acting" stimulants. Our ADHD drugs used to work an average of four hours. Now long-acting versions can help patients remain relatively symptom-free for up to twelve hours. One 2006 study showed that while 40 to 50 percent of those on short-acting medication were satisfied with their treatment, the numbers bump up to 70 percent for those taking the long-acting drugs. As a bonus, those of us with ADHD have a tough time remembering to take pills multiple times a day, so it's easy to see why long-acting stimulants have quickly become the standard of care.

One uniquely different, relatively new long-acting drug on the market is

Vyvanse. Approved in 2008, it is a stimulant that cannot be abused (i.e., snorted or injected). Its delivery system is different in that it is activated by an enzyme in the red blood cells in the gut. Because of this unique delivery system, it also lasts longer. While it advertises twelve to sixteen hours of efficacy, it averages being effective in a concentrated way for about ten hours. It's become one of the most popular drugs on the market because of its long-acting properties and because it is completely soluble, so it's easy to administer in beverage form to kids who don't like to take pills. It can be taken with or without food, giving parents options.

An even newer drug touting a long-acting and novel delivery system has the catchy name of Mydayis. Launched in 2017, this pill boasts a sixteen-hour cycle activated within your body in three steps—morning, noon, and evening.

Long-acting drugs are extremely popular, but when first trying medication it is advisable to use the short-acting stimulants until it can be determined that the drug can be well tolerated.

ADDICTION AND ABUSE

Spoiler alert! Taking a stimulant or stimulant-like drug early in life helps *prevent,* not promote, addiction later on. Since *80 percent of addictions* get started between the ages of thirteen and twenty-three, and since people with ADHD are far more prone to develop an addiction than the general population, and since taking stimulant medication *reduces* the risk of addiction later on, it makes a lot of sense to start a child on stimulant medication before age thirteen.

Addiction and abuse are understandably some of the main concerns cited by those reluctant to take an ADHD drug, and the concerns are valid. In fact, ADHD drugs are listed among the top drugs abused by high school and college students. It's important to note, though, that ADHD stimulant drugs are mainly used inappropriately by those not even diagnosed with ADHD. These "neurotypical" abusers use them to stay up to study, or mix them with other drugs of abuse, like alcohol and marijuana, to intensify the high, among other reasons only teenagers can come up with.

It is less common for those who have ADHD to purposely take far too much of a stimulant medication. Long-term studies found that those with ADHD who are successfully treated with stimulants become addicted to substances far less than the general population, and certainly less than the population who have ADHD and do not take stimulant medication.

On the flip side, teens who have ADHD and are not treated are five to ten times more likely to become addicted to substances. It is a myth that people come to psychiatrists to get the highest dose and greatest number of pills. Indeed, one of the biggest problems we encounter is that patients do not take the total prescribed dosage for the month. The tough part is keeping them on the medicine, not making sure they aren't angling for an overabundance of extra-strength medication. That being said, when people do go off stimulant medication, they can experience slight symptoms of withdrawal. This happens every evening, and the symptoms can be so mild as to be missed, or can lead to increasing tiredness, anxiety, aggression, or a variety of other presentations. Which leads us to a discussion of common side effects.

SIDE EFFECTS

Some of the most frequent side effects associated with ADHD medications are irritability, dry mouth, disruption of sleep, headaches, and a decrease in appetite. There can be an increase in heart rate and blood pressure over time (which are minimal), so some worry about how it will impact the heart in the long term. Recent studies have shown the effects are slim to none, but there are always warnings when taking medication. This is why it is extremely important to be closely monitored by your doctor when on a prescription, especially in the beginning stages.

Last but not least, there is a happy byproduct of treating ADHD with prescription medication: Proper diagnosis and treatment can not only help your ADHD but also be protective against secondary problems like anxiety and/or depression.

GENETIC TESTING TO AID IN SELECTING MEDICATION

The treatment of cancer gained spectacular results from studying patients' genes, from discovering biomarkers for various forms of cancer, and from planning treatment based upon a patient's genetic profile. Naturally, researchers started to look at genetic testing for diseases of the mind and the field of psychiatry. Indeed, for some time now, clinicians like us have been able to submit a sample of a patient's DNA—derived from saliva, blood, skin, or even hair—to a company that will assay the sample and provide a genetic analysis.

Patients and clinicians alike hoped that such an analysis could tell us what drug or medication to use. But in talking to the best experts we know, the verdict has consistently been "It's promising, but we're not there yet." So we do not routinely get genetic testing on our patients to guide our choice of medication unless the patient insists upon it. It certainly does no harm, other than that it can cost anywhere up to $2,000, depending on the test, the company, and the extent of one's health insurance coverage.

These tests will not tell you or your doctor exactly which drug will work best. This is the "there" we're not yet at, as much as we all would like to be. But these genetic tests can provide extremely valuable information on how rapidly you will metabolize a certain medication, which can help tremendously in dosing and in some cases prevent a disaster—if you lack a certain enzyme, for example.

We found one company we really like, called Tempus,[*2] based in Chicago. The man who founded it in 2015 did so because he was appalled at the lack of genetic data that doctors could draw upon to develop a treatment plan for his wife's cancer. So he set about building his own company to change that situation.

But then, in 2018, Tempus started looking into psychiatry as well as cancer testing. Most companies offer what's called "small panel sequencing," reporting on twelve to fifteen genes and correlating them with medications that might be prescribed.

Tempus stands out from the crowd because it uses what's called "whole exome sequencing." A strand of DNA contains *exons,* which are the coding sites—the sites that dictate the action—as well as *introns,* whose function is debated. Right now the intron seems to be a spectator to the action, but nature rarely creates spectators, so some essential function will likely be found. But we know for sure the exons matter a lot. Taken together, the exons form an *exome.*

Whole exome testing is important because in compiling it (coupled with the patient's personal history and family history, which Tempus also collects) biomarkers can appear in what at first seems like a vast field of irrelevant data. So Tempus wants to collect and test for the whole shebang.

By doing whole exome sequencing rather than the more common small panel sequencing, Tempus is not only laying a foundation for new discoveries, but also giving the patient and the doctor more information to work with.

You'd think that since you're getting more information, the cost would reflect that. Not so. Tempus seeks reimbursement from insurance companies for their test and has a robust financial assistance program to avoid undue financial burden on the patient. The majority of applicants qualify for a maximum out-of-pocket cost of no more than $100 for the test. So when the maximum you might pay is $100, with zero dollars being a distinct possibility, the risk of financial harm previously associated with testing is eliminated for many patients.

It seems to us that the time has come to at least consider using genetic testing routinely in prescribing medications.

THE MEDICAL ARSENAL AT A GLANCE

For a more complete rundown of stimulants and non-stimulants and outliers used to treat ADHD, we've included this helpful chart, originally printed in, and reprinted with the permission of, *ADDitude* magazine, a helpful resource for both clinicians and patients.

*1 Neither of us receives any funding from drug companies.

*2 Neither Dr. Hallowell nor Dr. Ratey receives any compensation from Tempus. Not even lunch!

ADHD Medication

MEDICATION	FORMULA-TION	COMPOUND	DURA-TION	DOSING CONSIDERA-TIONS
METHYLPHENIDATE				
Adhansia XR® (Adlon Therapeutics)	Extended-release capsule 25 mg, 35 mg, 45 mg. 55 mg, 70 mg, 85 mg	Capsule with multilayer beads; 20% immediate-release layer and 80% controlled-release layer	12 hours or more	Capsule may be opened and contents swallowed completely with applesauce
Aptensio XR® (Rhodes Pharmaceuticals)	Extended-release capsule 10 mg, 15 mg, 20 mg, 30 mg, 40 mg, 50 mg, 60 mg	Capsule with multilayer beads; 40% of dose in the immediate-release layer and 60% in the extended-release layer (2nd peak at 7–8 hrs)	12 hours	Capsule may be opened and contents swallowed completely with applesauce
Concerta® or generic[1] (Janssen and others)	Extended-release tablet 18 mg, 27 mg, 36 mg, 54 mg	Tablet with OROS osmotic pump technology; biphasic release with initial peak at 1 hr (22% of dose) and 78% gradual release over 9 hrs. Only Patriot version is authorized for substitution for brand at pharmacy.	12 hours	Must be swallowed whole; non-absorbable shell may be passed in stool
Cotempla XRODT™ (NEOS Therapeutics)	Extended-release orally disintegrating tablet 8.6 mg, 17.3 mg, 25.9 mg	Dissolving tablet with 25% immediate-release microparticles and 75% extended-release	12–13 hours	Grape-flavored; allow to dissolve in saliva
Daytrana® (Noven Therapeutics)	Transdermal patch 10 mg, 15 mg, 20 mg, 30 mg	Drug dispersed in adhesive layer; applied daily	9 hour wear-time	The time worn can be varied to control the duration of effects; monitor for skin rash or sensitivity. Discard patches appropriately. Slow onset of medication over initial six hours.

JORNAY PM™ (Ironshore Pharmaceuticals)	Delayed release— Extended release capsule 20mg, 40mg, 60mg, 80mg, 100mg	Dual-layer delexis delivery: outer layer delays release for up to 10 hours; inner layer controls daytime release	12–14 hours	Taken before going to sleep to provide early morning symptom control
Metadate CD® (UCB, Inc.)	Extended-release capsule 10 mg, 20 mg, 30 mg, 40 mg, 50 mg, 60 mg	Diffucaps capsule with 30% immediate-release beads and 70% delayed-release beads[*2]	8–10 hours	Capsule may be opened and contents swallowed completely with applesauce
Methylphenidate HCl (Lupin)	Chewable tablet 2.5 mg, 5 mg, 10 mg	Methylphenidate HCl	3–4 hours	Grape-flavored chewable tablet
Methylphenidate HCl (Mallinckrodt Pharmaceuticals)	Extended-release tablet[*3] 10 mg, 20 mg	Methylphenidate HCl	6–8 hours	Swallow whole; do not crush or chew
Methylin™ Liquid or generic (Shionogi Pharma and others)	Oral solution 5 mg/5 mL, 10 mg/5 mL	Methylphenidate HCl	3–4 hours	Colorless, grape-flavored liquid; store at room temperature
Quillichew ER™ (Tris Pharmaceuticals)	Extended-release chewable tablet 20 mg, 30 mg, 40 mg	30% of the dose is immediate-release and 70% extended-release	8 hours	Cherry-flavored; may be taken with or without food
Quillivant XR® (Tris Pharmaceuticals)	Extended-release oral suspension 25 mg/5 mL	20% of the dose is immediate-release and 80% extended-release	12 hours	Fruit-flavored; may be taken with or without food. Shake bottle for at least 10 seconds. May be stored at room temperature.
Ritalin® or generic (Novartis and others)	Short-acting, immediate-release tablet 5 mg, 10 mg, 20 mg	Methylphenidate HCl	3–4 hours	Abrupt onset and offset increase the number and severity of side effects
Ritalin LA® (Novartis)	Extended-release capsule 10	Capsule with Spheroidal Oral Drug Absorption	8–12 hours	Capsule may be opened and contents swallowed completely with applesauce

	mg, 20 mg, 30 mg, 40 mg, 60 mg	System (SODAS) technology; 50% immediate-release beads and 50% delayed-release (2nd peak 4 hrs later)[*4]		
Ritalin SR® (Novartis)	Sustained-release tablet 20 mg	Methylphenidate HCl	8 hours	Tablets should be swallowed whole, never crushed or chewed

DEXMETHYLPHENIDATE				
Focalin® or generic (Novartis and others)	Short-acting, immediate-release tablet[*5] 2.5 mg, 5 mg, 10 mg	Dexmethylphenidate Hydrochloride	4–6 hours	Isolated active dextroisomer; give approximately one-half methylphenidate dose
Focalin XR® or generic (Novartis and others)	Extended-release capsule 5 mg, 10 mg, 15 mg, 20 mg, 25 mg, 30 mg, 35 mg, 40 mg	Capsule with SODAS technology; 50% of the beads contained in the capsule are immediate-release and 50% are delayed-release[*6]	8–12 hours	Capsule may be opened and beads swallowed completely with applesauce

AMPHETAMINE				
Adzenys ER™ (Neos Therapeutics)	Extended-release oral suspension 1.25 mg/mL	50% immediate-release and 50% delayed-release particles	10–12 hours	Orange-flavored; may be taken with or without food. Shake bottle vigorously before dispensing the dose.
Adzenys XR-ODT™ (Neos Therapeutics)	Extended-release orally disintegrating tablet 3.1 mg, 6.3 mg, 9.4 mg, 12.5 mg, 15.7 mg, 18.8 mg	Dissolving tablet with 50% immediate-release and 50% delayed-release particles	10–12 hours	Allow tablet to dissolve in saliva
Dyanavel® XR (Tris Pharma)	Extended-release oral suspension 2.5 mg/mL	Oral solution with bubble gum flavor	13 hours	Bubble gum flavor; may be taken with or without food. Shake bottle before preparing the dose. May be stored at room temperature.

DEXTROAMPHETAMINE				
Dexedrine® or generic (Amedra Pharmaceuticals and others)	Short-acting tablet 5mg, 10 mg	Dextroamphetamine Sulfate	3–4 hours	Take first dose on awakening
Dexedrine ER® or generic (Amedra Pharmaceuticals and others)	Extended-release spansule 5 mg, 10mg, 15 mg	Dextroamphetamine Sulfate delivered in a sustained-release spansule. Initial dose released immediately, remaining medication released gradually.	5–10 hours	
ProCentra® or generic (Independence Pharma, Tris Pharma, and others)	Oral solution 5mg/5mL	Dextroamphetamine Sulfate	3–6 hours	Bubble gum flavor; may be taken with or without food. Shake bottle before preparing the dose. May be stored at room temperature.
Zenzedi® (Arbor Pharmaceuticals)	Immediate-release tablet 2.5 mg, 5 mg, 7.5 mg, 10 mg, 15 mg, 20 mg, 30 mg	Dextroamphetamine Sulfate	4–6 hours	Take first dose on awakening
METHAMPHETAMINE				
Desoxyn® or generic (Recordati Rare Diseases and others)	Immediate-release tablet 5 mg	Methamphetamine	4–6 hours	
MIXED AMPHETAMINE SALTS				
Adderall® or generic (CorePharma and others)	Short-acting, immediate-release tablet 5 mg, 7.5 mg, 10 mg, 12.5 mg, 15 mg, 20 mg, 30 mg	Dextroamphetamine Saccharate, Amphetamine Aspartate, Dextroamphetamine Sulfate, and Amphetamine Sulfate	4–6 hours	May be taken with or without food

Adderall® XR or generic (Takeda and others)	Extended-release capsule 5 mg, 10 mg, 15 mg, 20 mg, 25 mg, 30 mg	Capsule with Microtrol delivery system: 50% immediate-release and 50% delayed-release beads[7]	10–12 hours	Capsule may be opened and beads swallowed whole with applesauce
Mydayis® (Takeda)	Long-acting capsule 12.5 mg, 25 mg, 37.5 mg, 50 mg	Long-acting, triple-bead, mixed-amphetamine salts formulation	14–16 hours	Capsule may be opened and beads swallowed whole with applesauce
AMPHETAMINE SULFATE				
Evekeo® (Arbor Pharmaceuticals)	Immediate-release tablet 5 mg, 10 mg	50% dextroamphetamine and 50% levoamphetamine	4–6 hours	
LISDEXAMFETAMINE				
Vyvanse® (Takeda)	Long-acting capsule 10 mg, 20 mg, 30 mg, 40 mg, 50 mg, 60 mg, 70 mg	Lisdexamfetamine Dimesylate; peaks in 3.5 hrs[8]	10–13 hours	Capsule may be opened and contents dissolved in water, yogurt, or orange juice; use immediately after dissolving
Vyvanse® (Takeda)	Chewable tablet 10 mg, 20 mg, 30mg, 40 mg, 50 mg, 60 mg	Lisdexamfetamine Dimesylate; peaks in 3.5 hrs[9]	10–13 hours	Strawberry flavored; may be taken with or without food
ATOMOXETINE				
Strattera® or generic (Lilly and others)	Long-acting capsule 10 mg, 18 mg, 25 mg, 40 mg, 60 mg, 80 mg, 100 mg	All-day atomoxetine	24 hours	Selective norepinephrine inhibitor. Starts working in a few days to one week, but may take several weeks to achieve full effect. Swallow capsule whole; powder is irritating. Dose is commonly divided in two to lower side effects.
CLONIDINE				
Kapvay® or	Extended-	Clonidine	24 hours	Swallow tablet whole

generic clonidine ER (Advanz Pharmaceuticals and others)	release tablet 0.1 mg, 0.2 mg	Hydrochloride		
GUANFACINE				
Intuniv™ or generic (Takeda and others)	Extended-release tablet 1 mg, 2 mg, 3 mg, 4 mg	Guanfacine	24 hours	Swallow tablet whole; a high-fat meal may increase absorption and lead to toxicity. FDA-approved for doses up to 7 mg.
BUPROPION				
Wellbutrin XL® (Valeant Pharmaceuticals)	Extended-release tablet 150 mg, 300 mg	Bupropion HCL	24 hours	Low efficacy; takes eight weeks to fully develop benefits. IR dosed three times a day; SR dosed two times a day; XL dosed once a day.

Skip Notes

*1 Note that most of the formulations that are marketed as "generic Concerta" are not reliable and have been downgraded from AB status to BX ("cannot be substituted for the brand name by the pharmacy"). As of September 2019, patients should accept only the Patriot generic, which is "authorized" by the brand name maker.

*2 Administration with a high-fat meal may affect the rate of absorption of some medications, but it has no significant effect on the total amount of the medication that is absorbed.

*3 Administration with a high-fat meal may affect the rate of absorption of some medications, but it has no significant effect on the total amount of the medication that is absorbed.

*4 Administration with a high-fat meal may affect the rate of absorption of some medications, but it has no significant effect on the total amount of the medication that is absorbed.

*5 Administration with a high-fat meal may affect the rate of absorption of some medications, but it has no significant effect on the total amount of the medication that is absorbed.

*6 Administration with a high-fat meal may affect the rate of absorption of some medications, but it has no significant effect on the total amount of the medication that is absorbed.

*7 Administration with a high-fat meal may affect the rate of absorption of some medications, but it has no significant effect on the total amount of the medication that is absorbed.

*8 Administration with a high-fat meal may affect the rate of absorption of some medications, but it has no significant effect on the total amount of the medication that is absorbed.

*9 Administration with a high-fat meal may affect the rate of absorption of some medications, but it has no significant effect on the total amount of the medication that is absorbed.

CHAPTER 9

Putting It All Together: Find Your Feel and Make It Real

f you have ADHD, variable attention stimulus trait (VAST), a race car brain with bicycle brakes, or whatever term you've settled on for this blessed and cursed kind of brain, it's likely you've reached this page without having read the entire book. That's okay, we certainly understand; we know that people like us tend to skip to the end to find the punch line, that we like to put the cart before the proverbial horse.

Let us fill you in briefly: What the cart contained was a lot of stories, explanations, suggestions, and science on how to turn the kind of brain we have into an extraordinary asset while preventing it from becoming the terrible curse it can sometimes be. ADHD and VAST have brought such shame and pain to so many who don't deserve it that we're passionate about using what we know and doing all that we can to end that shame and pain.

ADHD was totally misunderstood for so very, very long. Tragically, terribly misunderstood. This led to the sadistic and systematic betrayal of innocent children, punishing them for what they could not control, and the wholesale wasting of the talent of generations of adults. For far too long, it was considered okay to call those of us with ADHD imbeciles, morons, and idiots. Based on IQ, those were actual diagnostic terms in medical textbooks well into the 1960s. Who wouldn't want to skip to the end of *that*?

But why did you pick up the book at all? What were you looking for? Were you hoping for a happy ending?

If so, you've come to the right place! We can give you that happy ending. Not an ending, actually, but a point of demarcation, because finally we're getting it right in some places, most of the time. Finally, the world is catching on that our issue isn't laziness or disrespect or self-indulgence. No, our neural functioning is slightly but meaningfully different from that of the "neurotypicals" in the population. There is a sometimes glitchy connection between our task-positive network and the default mode network in our brains. And our cerebellum—another area of the brain—is often a little off balance and in need of strengthening. In other words, the science is proving that we aren't just trying to be difficult; we're really having a difficult time inside. We also know that connection to others, identifying our strengths and focusing on them instead of our weaknesses, setting up systems of structure in our environments, getting exercise, and taking medication all really help with these glitches and imbalances.

The other thing the world is starting to see is the tremendous potential— creativity, entrepreneurial spirit, energy—of people with this condition. We see the amazing accomplishments of people with ADHD every day in our practices; as successful authors and clinicians with ADHD, we see this in ourselves, too!

Now it's time for all of us to join together and apply what we know so the doors of opportunity, of creativity, and of understanding will open to people of all ages with ADHD. We've written this book to show you where you might find the keys to those doors.

While each chapter in this book highlights one finding, strategy, or treatment to fit into your ADHD-coping puzzle, ultimately we know that you will need to put the pieces together in your own unique way. If you play golf (and even if you don't), consider this conversational exchange between Dr. Hallowell and his brother-in-law, Chris, who is a golf pro in Virginia. Hidden therein lies great advice for not only surviving but *thriving* with ADHD, which we'll explain.

CHRIS, calmly: Ned, you just need to find your feel and make it real. And remember that the key to putting is not caring if the ball goes in the hole.

DR. HALLOWELL (known as Ned), sputtering and incredulous: But, Chris, I'm *praying* the ball goes in the hole. How could I *possibly* not care?

CHRIS, ever the Yoda-like sage: You'll putt better when you learn how.

This is, essentially, the advice this book has been offering throughout. We want to help you find your feel and make it real. And we want to keep you out of the success/failure trap that prevents so many people from achieving happiness.

Just as everyone has their own style of putting, their own unique feel for that devilish art, so each of us has our own style of living life, our own feel for doing all we do. Look at your style, your feel. Is it truly yours or are you imitating someone else's? Most everything we do is part imitation, but what makes each of us unique is what we add in on our own to create our individuality, our special sauce, our style. Or as Dr. Hallowell wrote in his poem to his five-year-old daughter, "No brain is the same, no brain is the best, each brain finds its own special way."

We've offered what we believe to be the best techniques all people with ADHD can use, but whether you use them or how you use them—that you have to personalize. Find *your* feel. What feels right for one of us won't necessarily feel right for you.

At the risk of alienating anyone who has never played golf, we need to extend this golf-as-life metaphor just a little further. If you don't play, you've missed out on enjoying the feeling of hitting a perfect golf shot. Let us walk you through it: You step up to the ball, you set your stance, and then you swing. When it's right, you don't even feel the club hit the ball. You just swing through it and, replacing brute force with beautifully balanced torque (when you do it right), you launch that dimpled devil into flight. It quickly becomes a fading dot, a shooting star, against the blue or cloudy sky.

The swing finished, the mechanical part of your performance complete, you track the ball with mounting pride as it does what you'd hoped it would do, what you dream it will do whenever you imagine playing golf, and your heart fills with the joy of having made a perfect shot, having beaten golf at its own game and entropy to boot, having prevailed over the zillion factors that could have gone wrong and turned your drive into a flub.

But no flub this time. This time you got it right. You nailed it. This time you achieved the feeling you always seek but rarely find, the feeling of having prevailed in the contest with whatever makes things go wrong, the feeling of mastery over a foe you know will likely strike back hard next time. But this time, this one fine time, you brought that foe down to defeat in one graceful and glorious *whooosh*.

Okay, buddy, you say to yourself, *do it again.* How those words taunt through eternity. *Do it again.* To do it again, consistently, that's the dream we all share but few of us achieve.

This is where the part about not caring if the ball drops into the hole comes into play. Chris's don't-care advice may seem counterintuitive, but we have learned it's spot-on. It doesn't mean you're blasé. It just means your focus is on the moment, not the outcome.

We leave you with our hope that you will stay in the game and focus on the moment. Try to appreciate how silly and shallow an overemphasis on winning truly is, and how shortsighted and unimaginative it is to allow defeat to define you. Try to remember that life's great reward, its greatest joy, lies in the game itself—the trying to figure it out, the trying new ways to do so. Revel in it. Suffer in it. Stick with it as if your life depends upon it, because it does. Work at forever finding your feel and making it real. Cherish the great shot, for sure. Nothing beats it. But, oddly, cherish the flub just as much. It makes you want to try again and gives you something to shoot for. And, to mangle the famous saying, flubbing reminds you what it is to be human: to make mistakes.

Each of us finds a different way; there is no one right way. But what a liberating message it is for us all to know that no brain is the best, and each of us has the magnificent, lifelong chance to find our own brain's special way.

channeled Elvin Semrad beautifully for me and got me started sitting with patients.

Above all, and always, my wife of thirty-two years, Sue, and our children, Lucy, Jack, and Tucker. They add such sunshine, energy, and love to my life every day that I can never thank them enough.

—EDWARD (NED) HALLOWELL

I, too, take pleasure in thanking the people who have been instrumental in getting this book started and completed. Grateful acknowledgment goes to our editor, Marnie Cochran, who has done so much to hone the book into its current form. She has been tireless and exacting in corralling our thoughts and focusing our energies.

I'm also deeply indebted to Ned Hallowell, my student, now teacher, and treasured friend over these many years. He provided the spark to take on the challenge of writing a new book together and once again penned his thoughts, and mine, to bring us this latest achievement.

Thanks also to my mentors of the past, George Vaillant, Allan Hobson, and Richard Shader, who were not put off by my ADHD enthusiasm but encouraged and guided me to "go for it." And to my business partner and wonderful friend Ben Lopez, who taught me to reach beyond the norm. As always, I am also eternally beholden to my patients over the years, who have shared their lives with me and taught me so much.

Finally, I gratefully acknowledge my wife, Alicia Ulrich, who has been a partner in interviewing and thinking about my parts of the manuscript, along with being a true and honest sounding board. It is her love, and the love of my daughters, Jessie and Kathryn, and grandchildren, Gracie and Callum, that makes everything I do worthwhile.

—JOHN RATEY

Appendix A

THE DIAGNOSTIC AND STATISTICAL MANUAL OF MENTAL DISORDERS DEFINITION OF AND CRITERIA FOR ADHD (ABRIDGED)

People with ADHD show a persistent pattern of inattention and/or hyperactivity—impulsivity that interferes with functioning or development:

1. Inattention: Six or more symptoms of inattention for children up to age 16, or five or more for adolescents 17 and older and adults; symptoms of inattention have been present for at least 6 months, and they are inappropriate for developmental level:

    -   Often fails to give close attention to details or makes careless mistakes in schoolwork, at work, or with other activities.
    -   Often has trouble holding attention on tasks or play activities.
    -   Often does not seem to listen when spoken to directly.
    -   Often does not follow through on instructions and fails to finish schoolwork, chores, or duties in the workplace (e.g., loses focus, becomes sidetracked).
    -   Often has trouble organizing tasks and activities.
    -   Often avoids, dislikes, or is reluctant to do tasks that require mental effort over a long period of time (such as schoolwork or homework).
    -   Often loses things necessary for tasks and activities (e.g., school materials, pencils, books, tools, wallets, keys, paperwork, eyeglasses, mobile telephones).
    -   Is often easily distracted.

    ◦ Is often forgetful in daily activities.

2. Hyperactivity and Impulsivity: Six or more symptoms of hyperactivity-impulsivity for children up to age 16, or five or more for adolescents 17 and older and adults; symptoms of hyperactivity-impulsivity have been present for at least 6 months to an extent that is disruptive and inappropriate for the person's developmental level:

    ◦ Often fidgets with or taps hands or feet, or squirms in seat.

    ◦ Often leaves seat in situations when remaining seated is expected.

    ◦ Often runs about or climbs in situations where it is not appropriate (adolescents or adults may be limited to feeling restless).

    ◦ Often is unable to play or take part in leisure activities quietly.

    ◦ Is often "on the go," acting as if "driven by a motor."

    ◦ Often talks excessively.

    ◦ Often blurts out an answer before a question has been completed.

    ◦ Often has trouble waiting his/her turn.

    ◦ Often interrupts or intrudes on others (e.g., butts into conversations or games).

In addition, the following conditions must be met:

- Several inattentive or hyperactive-impulsive symptoms were present before age 12 years.
- Several symptoms are present in two or more settings (such as at home, school, or work; with friends or relatives; in other activities).
- There is clear evidence that the symptoms interfere with, or reduce the quality of, social, school, or work functioning.
- The symptoms are not better explained by another mental disorder (such as a mood disorder, anxiety disorder, dissociative disorder, or a personality disorder). The symptoms do not happen only during the course of schizophrenia or another psychotic disorder.

Based on the types of symptoms, three kinds (presentations) of ADHD can occur:

- Combined Presentation: if enough symptoms of both criteria inattention and hyperactivity-impulsivity were present for the past 6 months
- Predominantly Inattentive Presentation: if enough symptoms of inattention, but not hyperactivity-impulsivity, were present for the past six months
- Predominantly Hyperactive-Impulsive Presentation: if enough symptoms of hyperactivity-impulsivity, but not inattention, were present for the past six months.

Because symptoms can change over time, the presentation may change over time as well.

DIAGNOSING ADHD IN ADULTS

ADHD often lasts into adulthood. To diagnose ADHD in adults and adolescents age 17 or older, only 5 symptoms are needed instead of the 6 needed for younger children. Symptoms might look different at older ages. For example, in adults, hyperactivity may appear as extreme restlessness or wearing others out with their activity.

Appendix B

A COMPENDIUM OF RESOURCES

EDWARD M. HALLOWELL, M.D.

www.drhallowell.com

Provides resources containing the latest information and treatment recommendations on ADD/ADHD for people of all ages, plus advice on parenting, academics, work/life/home concerns, relationships, and more.

TREATMENT CENTERS FOR PEOPLE OF ALL AGES WITH ADHD

THE HALLOWELL CENTERS

www.drhallowell.com

Each Hallowell Center practices the Hallowell Strength-Based comprehensive evaluation and innovative multidisciplinary treatment for ADHD and other mental health concerns, rooted in the practices, philosophy, and writings of Dr. Hallowell.

California

HALLOWELL TODARO ADHD CENTER PALO ALTO

www.hallowelltodaro.com

650-446-4900

Rooted in Dr. Hallowell's Strength-Based approach, this practice is interdisciplinary, like the other Hallowell Centers. Dr. Hallowell teamed up with an extraordinary clinician, Lesley Todaro, LMFTA, CDPT, to found this center.

HALLOWELL CENTER SAN FRANCISCO

www.hallowellsfo.com

415-967-0061

Comprehensive evaluation and multidisciplinary, innovative Hallowell Strength-Based treatments and integrative approaches for ADHD, depression, anxiety, relationship/career/education/life issues, and other mental health concerns.

Massachusetts

THE HALLOWELL CENTER BOSTON METROWEST

www.drhallowellsudbury.com

978-287-0810

This is the first Hallowell Center, opened in 1996. Dr. Hallowell splits his private practice time between his center in Boston MetroWest and New York. The Boston facility has a staff of more than twenty clinicians who specialize in the Hallowell Strength-Based treatment of ADHD in children and adults.

New York
Manhattan and Surrounding Areas

THE HALLOWELL CENTER NYC

www.hallowellcenter.org

212-799-7777

Dr. Hallowell splits his private practice time between his centers in Boston MetroWest and New York. The New York facility has a staff of more than twenty clinicians who specialize in the Hallowell Strength-Based treatment of ADHD in children and adults.

Washington
Kirkland and Seattle

HALLOWELL-TODARO ADHD CENTER

www.hallowelltodarocenter.org

206-420-7345

Rooted in Dr. Hallowell's Strength-Based approach, this practice is interdisciplinary, like the other Hallowell Centers. Dr. Hallowell teamed up with an extraordinary clinician, Lesley Todaro, LMFTA, CDPT, to found this center. Ms. Todaro runs the center with her team of clinicians and administrators.

Centers Using Dr. Hallowell's Strength-Based Approach

Massachusetts
Hingham

CENTER FOR INTEGRATIVE COUNSELING AND WELLNESS

www.centerforintegrativecounselingandwellness.com

781-749-9227

Email: info@CenterforIntegrativeCounselingandWellness.com

The center offers a range of services from traditional psychotherapy and psychiatry to holistic approaches, including Dr. Hallowell's Strength-Based approach to treating ADHD, all available in one convenient location.

SUPPORT, EDUCATION, AND ADVOCACY ORGANIZATIONS

The organizations listed below offer information and support to those in need. Call to locate an office or support group near you, as well as to obtain a list of their individual publications and membership information.

ADHD Organizations

A.D.D. RESOURCE CENTER

www.addrc.org

646-205-8080

Proven, practical program and services for dealing with ADD/ADHD.

AMERICAN ACADEMY OF CHILD AND ADOLESCENT PSYCHIATRY

www.aacap.org

202-966-7300

Though not specifically an ADHD-oriented organization, child and adolescent psychiatrists can be an enormous help in supporting you or your child.

AMERICAN PSYCHOLOGICAL ASSOCIATION (APA)

www.apa.org/topics/adhd/index.aspx

800-374-2721

The APA is not specifically focused on ADHD issues, but it is the leading scientific and professional organization representing psychology in the United States, with more than 117,500 researchers, educators, clinicians, consultants, and students as its members.

ATTENTION DEFICIT DISORDER ASSOCIATION (ADDA)

www.add.org

800-939-1019

Provides information, resources, and networking opportunities to help adults with ADHD lead better lives.

CENTER FOR MANAGEMENT OF ADHD RESOURCES

Children's Hospital of Philadelphia

www.chop.edu/centers-programs/center-management-adhd/health-resources

800-879-2467

Provides ADHD resources for educators, parents, caregivers, and adults.

CENTER FOR PARENT INFORMATION AND RESOURCES (CPIR)

www.parentcenterhub.org/

Email: malizo@spannj.org

CPIR serves as a central resource of information and products to the community of Parent Training Information (PTI) Centers and the Community Parent Resource Centers (CPRCs) so that they can focus their efforts on serving families of children with disabilities.

CHADD (CHILDREN AND ADULTS WITH ATTENTION DEFICIT DISORDER)

www.CHADD.org

301-306-7070

CHADD provides support, training, education, and advocacy and works to ensure that those with ADHD reach their inherent potential. As home to the

National Resource Center on ADHD, funded by the U.S. Centers for Disease Control and Prevention, CHADD is the most trusted source of reliable, science-based information regarding current medical research and ADHD management.

CHILD MIND INSTITUTE

www.childmind.org

212-308-3118

The Child Mind Institute is an independent national nonprofit dedicated to transforming the lives of children and families struggling with mental health and learning disorders.

EYE TO EYE

www.eyetoeyenational.org

212-537-4429, 628-400-4106

Founded and run by David Flink, Eye to Eye provides mentors for high school and college students who have learning differences.

HEALTHYCHILDREN.ORG

www.healthychildren.org/English/health-issues/conditions/adhd/Pages/Understanding-ADHD.aspx

Provides information and resources for parents on ADHD.

NATIONAL RESEARCH CENTER ON ADHD

www.help4adhd.org

800-233-4050

The nation's clearinghouse for evidence-based information on ADHD.

Learning Disabilities Organizations

COUNCIL FOR EXCEPTIONAL CHILDREN (CEC)

www.cec.sped.org

703-620-3660

A nonprofit organization with seventeen specialized divisions. DLD (see below) is the division dedicated to learning disabilities. It provides free information and holds conferences.

COUNCIL FOR LEARNING DISABILITIES (CLD)

www.cldinternational.org

913-491-1011

CLD, an international organization composed of professionals who represent diverse disciplines, is committed to enhancing the education and quality of life for individuals with learning disabilities across the life span.

DIVISION FOR LEARNING DISABILITIES (DLD)

www.teachingld.org

DLD is an international professional organization consisting of teachers, psychologists, clinicians, administrators, higher education professionals, parents, and others.

HELPGUIDE

www.helpguide.org/articles/add-adhd/attention-deficit-disorder-adhd-parenting-tips.htm

Comprehensive guide for resources for mental, emotional, and social health.

INTERNATIONAL DYSLEXIA ASSOCIATION (IDA)

www.interdys.org

410-296-0232, 800-222-3123

Email: info@interdys.org

IDA is the oldest organization dedicated to the study and treatment of dyslexia. The society has more than forty branches throughout the United States and Canada that offer informational meetings and support groups. Referrals are made for persons seeking resources.

LEARNING DISABILITIES ASSOCIATION OF AMERICA (LDA)

www.ldaamerica.org

412-341-1515

Email: info@ldaamerica.org

LDA believes that every person with learning disabilities can be successful at school, at work, in relationships, and in the community, given the right opportunities.

MENTAL HEALTH AMERICA (MHA)

www.mentalhealthamerica.net

MHA is dedicated to addressing the needs of those living with mental illness and to promoting the overall mental health of all Americans.

NATIONAL CENTER FOR LEARNING DISABILITIES (NCLD)

www.ncld.org

Founded in 1977, NCLD provides resources to improve the lives of children and adults nationwide with learning and attention issues, by empowering parents and young adults, transforming schools, and advocating for equal rights and opportunities.

NATIONAL INSTITUTE FOR LEARNING DEVELOPMENT (NILD)

www.nild.org

757-423-8646

Since 1973, NILD has developed its own individualized educational therapy to build competence and confidence in all learners, which includes a special form of tutoring, combined with exercises that stimulate certain parts of the brain. NILD has six hundred active therapists in thirty-five states and sixteen countries.

PARENT TO PARENT USA

www.p2pusa.org

Provides emotional and informational support for families of children who have special needs.

UNDERSTOOD

www.understood.org

Email: support@understood.org

Understood is a free online resource and community supporting millions of parents of kids with learning and attention issues by offering personalized recommendations, free daily access to experts, and a safe community. Understood was created by fifteen nonprofit partners in October 2014 to empower parents to help their kids thrive in school and in life.

Organizations Devoted to Disorders Related to ADHD

DEPRESSION AND BIPOLAR SUPPORT ALLIANCE (DBSA)

www.dbsalliance.org

800-826-3632

DBSA provides hope, help, support, and education to improve the lives of people who have mood disorders.

FEDERATION FOR CHILDREN WITH SPECIAL NEEDS

www.fcsn.org

617-236-7210, 800-331-0688

Email: fcsninfo@fcsn.org

Provides information, support, and assistance to parents of children with disabilities, their professional partners, and their communities.

JUVENILE BIPOLAR RESEARCH FOUNDATION

https://www.jbrf.org/

914-468-1297

Email: info@jbrf.org

Promotes and supports scientific research focused on the cause of and treatments for bipolar disorder in children.

NATIONAL ALLIANCE FOR THE MENTALLY ILL (NAMI)

www.nami.org

703-524-7600, 800-950-6264

NAMI, the nation's largest grassroots mental health organization, is dedicated to building better lives for the millions of Americans affected by mental illness.

TOURETTE ASSOCIATION OF AMERICA

www.tsa-usa.org

718-224-2999

Email: ts@tsa-usa.org

Offers resources and referrals to help people and their families cope with the problems that accompany Tourette syndrome.

Laws, Accommodations, and Employment Resources

ASSOCIATION ON HIGHER EDUCATION AND DISABILITY (AHEAD)

www.ahead.org

704-947-7779

AHEAD is a professional membership organization for individuals involved in the development of policy and in the provision of quality services to meet the needs of persons with disabilities involved in all areas of higher education.

EQUAL EMPLOYMENT OPPORTUNITY COMMISSION (EEOC)

www.eeoc.gov

202-663-4900

Email: info@eeoc.gov

Provides information on employment issues, federal laws, and discrimination.

JOB ACCOMMODATION NETWORK

www.jan.wvu.edu

800-526-7234

Email: jan@askjan.org

A free consulting service that provides information about job accommodations, the Americans with Disabilities Act (ADA), and the employability of people with disabilities.

OFFICE FOR CIVIL RIGHTS—OCR (U.S. DEPARTMENT OF EDUCATION)

www2.ed.gov/policy/landing.jhtml?src=pn

800-872-5327

OCR ensures equal access to education and promotes educational excellence throughout the nation through enforcement of civil rights. Contact OCR for Section 504–related issues.

Magazines, Newsletters, Podcasts, and Radio

***ADDITUDE* MAGAZINE**

www.additudemag.com

888-762-8475

Email: additude@additudemag.com

National bimonthly magazine for the ADHD community. Dr. Hallowell writes a regular column for this magazine.

THE ADHD REPORT BY RUSSELL A. BARKLEY, PH.D.

www.russellbarkley.org/newsletter.html

In 1993, Dr. Barkley founded *The ADHD Report* with Guilford Publications. This bimonthly newsletter is designed for clinicians and knowledgeable parents to provide them with the latest scientific information on ADHD. It contains insights and cutting-edge techniques of today's leading authorities on ADHD. Dr. Barkley is one of the pioneers in the field of ADHD.

ATTENTION MAGAZINE

www.chadd.org/membership/attention-magazine.aspx

Published quarterly, this publication is available with CHADD membership.

ATTENTION TALK RADIO

www.attentiontalkradio.com

The leading site for self-help Internet radio shows focusing on ADHD, including managing symptoms of attention deficit hyperactivity disorder. Target audience is adults with ADHD and adults who have children with ADHD.

DISTRACTION PODCAST

www.distractionpodcast.com

844-552-6663

Email: connect@distractionpodcast.com

Dr. Hallowell hosts a twice-weekly podcast called *Distraction*, which explores how we are driven to distraction and offers coping strategies for managing ADHD, technology, your crazy-busy life, and more. It can be downloaded and subscribed to on iTunes, Google Play Music, Stitcher, or the Distraction website.

Coaching Resources

ADDA COACH REGISTER

www.add.org/professional-directory

Listing of ADHD coaches throughout the United States, Canada, and Puerto

Rico.

ADD COACH ACADEMY

www.ADDCA.com

800-915-7702

Email: info@addca.com

Founded by David Giwerc, a pioneer in the coaching field. Great resource for finding a coach or becoming a coach.

ADD CONSULTS

www.addconsults.com

800-615-9786

Email: terry@addconsults.com

Helps women with ADHD get unstuck and on track. Provides private, personal ADHD consultations, both nationally and internationally, via email.

AMERICAN COACHING ASSOCIATION

www.americoach.org

610-825-8572

ACA's mission is to link people who want coaching with people who do coaching, to acquaint the general public with the concept of coaching, and to provide coaches with training, supervision, and a professional community.

BLUBERYL

www.bluberyl.com

978-225-0625

Email: info@bluberyl.com

BLUBERYL is a strength-based productivity and executive function coaching company that helps students and adults recognize and make the most of their own learning styles and preferences. BLUBERYL's proprietary programs and products teach clients how to become more organized and efficient at home, in school, and in their careers.

DIG COACHING PRACTICE

www.digcoaching.com/

813-837-8084

Email: jeff@digcoaching.com

Jeff Copper is an accredited, certified ADHD coach who helps others to overcome information overload, chronic disorganization, time blindness, procrastination, and all the ADHD symptoms related to self-regulation, impulsivity, distractibility, and other issues that may hinder one's advancement. Jeff specializes in working with adults, college students, and entrepreneurs.

IMPACT ADHD

www.impactadhd.com

888-535-6507

Email: theteam@impactadhd.com

Provides coaching, parenting programs, and resources for parents raising ADHD kids.

PTS COACHING: ADHD TRAINING, EDUCATION, AND SUPPORT

www.PTScoaching.com

516-802-0593

Email: info@PTScoaching.com

Creating pathways to success for parents, teachers, and students.

LESLIE ROUCER, COACH THERAPIST

www.addadults.net

561-706-1274

Email: leslie@addadults.net

Specializing in adult ADHD.

NANCY SNELL

www.nancysnell.com

212-517-6488

Certified professional business/ADHD coach, NYC, helping adults with productivity, business, and ADHD coaching since 2003.

ADHD Educational Materials

ADD WAREHOUSE

www.addwarehouse.com

800-233-9273

Email: websales@addwarehouse.com

Mail-order and online catalog of resources on ADHD, oppositional defiant disorder, Asperger's syndrome, autism, Tourette syndrome, and learning problems. It offers a wide variety of books, videos, and other resource materials.

Additional Web Resources

HABYTS

www.habyts.com

Email: contact@habyts.com

Habyts helps families build good habits for life, including helping parents manage screen time and motivate their kids to do chores and homework.

LD ONLINE

www.ldonline.org

LD OnLine seeks to help children and adults reach their full potential by providing accurate and up-to-date information and advice about learning disabilities and ADHD.

PSYCHOLOGY TODAY

www.psychologytoday.com/us

This long-running publication offers the best online directory of therapists, psychologists, and counselors and the latest news from the world of psychology, from behavioral research to practical guidance on relationships and mental health, including addiction.

SUGGESTED READINGS

For Children Who Have ADHD

Dendy, Chris A. Zeigler, and Alex Zeigler. *A Bird's-Eye View of Life with ADD and ADHD: Advice from Young Survivors.* Cedar Bluff, AL: Cherish the Children, 2003. (Written for teens by twelve teens and a young adult.)

Hallowell, Edward M., M.D. *A Walk in the Rain with a Brain*. New York: Regan Books/HarperCollins, 2004. An illustrated children's story (for ages four to twelve), the moral of which is that the words "smart" and "stupid" mean very little; what matters is finding what you love, then doing it. As Manfred the brain says in the story, "No brain is the same, no brain is the best, each brain finds its own special way."

Lowry, Mark, and Martha Bolton. *Piper's Night Before Christmas*. West Monroe, LA: Howard Publishing, 1998. This is the first in a series of four books; the others are *Nighttime Is Just Daytime with Your Eyes Closed* (1999), *Piper Steals the Show* (2000), and *Piper's Twisted Tale* (2001). Having grown up with ADHD, Mark Lowry readily identifies with the character in his books, Piper the Hyperactive Mouse. Mark is a multitalented artist who is a comedian, singer, and songwriter, as well as co-author of these children's books. Each book comes with a CD of Mark narrating the story.

Mooney, Jonathan, and David Cole. *Learning Outside the Lines*. New York: Touchstone, 2000. Two Ivy League students with learning disabilities and ADHD give you the tools for academic success and educational revolution.

Moss, Deborah. *Shelley, the Hyperactive Turtle*. Bethesda, MD: Woodbine House, 1989. The delightful story of a bright young turtle who is not like all the other turtles. Shelley moves like a rocket and is unable to sit still for even the shortest periods of time.

For Parents of Children Who Have ADHD

Barkley, Russell A., Ph.D. *Taking Charge of ADHD: The Complete, Authoritative Guide for Parents*. New York: Guilford Press, 2000. A parent resource incorporating the most current information on ADHD and its treatment.

Braaten, Ellen, and Brian Willoughby. *Bright Kids Who Can't Keep Up*. New York: Guilford Press, 2014. Filled with vivid stories and examples of kids and teens who struggle with an area of cognitive functioning called "processing speed," this crucial resource demystifies processing speed and shows how to help kids (ages five to eighteen) catch up in this key area of development.

Brooks, Robert, Ph.D., and Sam Goldstein, Ph.D. *Raising Resilient Children: Fostering Strength, Hope, and Optimism in Your Child.* New York: McGraw-Hill/Contemporary Books, 2002. This book explains how to help children become emotionally and mentally strong to face the challenges of modern life.

Flink, David. *Thinking Differently.* New York: HarperCollins, 2014. An innovative, comprehensive guide—the first of its kind—to help parents understand and accept learning disabilities in their children, offering tips and strategies for successfully advocating on their behalf and helping them become their own best advocates.

Galinsky, Ellen. *Mind in the Making: The Seven Essential Life Skills Every Child Needs.* New York: HarperStudio, 2010. This book presents groundbreaking advice based on the latest research on child development.

Goldrich, Cindy. *8 Keys to Parenting Children with ADHD.* New York: W. W. Norton, 2015. Based on the author's seven-session workshop entitled "Calm and Connected: Parenting Kids with ADHD," this book focuses on developing and strengthening effective interpersonal skills in both parents and children as a way to improve conflict resolution.

Greene, Ross, Ph.D. *The Explosive Child.* New York: HarperCollins, 1998. A practical approach to treating spirited children. Dr. Greene explains that the difficulties of these children stem from brain-based deficits in the ability to be flexible and to handle frustration.

Hallowell, Edward M., M.D. *The Childhood Roots of Adult Happiness.* New York: Ballantine, 2003. A succinct, practical, evidence-based guide for parents on how to raise children in a way that will maximize the chances of their becoming happy, successful adults, whether or not they have ADHD.

Hallowell, Edward M., M.D., and Peter Jensen. *Superparenting for ADD: An Innovative Approach to Raising Your Distracted Child.* New York: Ballantine, 2008. *Superparenting* shows you how to unwrap the wonderful, surprising gifts of ADHD and turn what is too often labeled a lifelong disability into a lifelong blessing.

Jensen, Peter S., M.D. *Making the System Work for Your Child with ADHD.* New York: Guilford Press, 2004.

Kenney, Lynne, and Wendy Young. *Bloom: 50 Things to Say, Think, and Do with Anxious, Angry, and Over-the-Top-Kids.* Boca Raton, FL: HCI Press, 2015. Written for parents with anxious, angry, and over-the-top kids, *Bloom* is a brain-based approach to parenting all children.

Krauss, Elaine, and Diane Dempster. *Parenting ADHD Now! Easy Intervention Strategies to Empower Kids with ADHD.* New York: Althea Press, 2016. This book is packed with helpful real-life, hands-on tips and tricks to help you parent your child with ADHD.

Morin, Amanda. *The Everything Parent's Guide to Special Education: A Complete Step-by-Step Guide to Advocating for Your Child with Special Needs.* Avon, MA: Adams Media, 2014. This valuable handbook gives you the tools you need to navigate the complex world of special education and services.

———. *The Everything Kids' Learning Activities Book: 145 Entertaining Activities and Learning Games for Kids.* Avon, MA: Adams Media, 2013.

Silver, Larry, M.D. *Dr. Larry Silver's Advice to Parents on ADHD.* New York: Three Rivers Press, 1999. This resource addresses the subjects all parents wonder about when they suspect their child has ADHD: causes, signs to look for, getting an accurate diagnosis, latest information on medications and other treatments.

Volpitta, Donna M., and Joel David Haber, Ph.D. *The Resilience Formula: A Guide to Proactive, Not Reactive, Parenting.* Chester, PA: Widener, 2012. The Resilience Formula is a plan for proactive parenting—parenting that teaches resilience to children through everyday challenges.

Wilens, Timothy E., M.D. *Straight Talk About Psychiatric Medications for Kids.* 4th ed. New York: Guilford Press, 2016. With numerous real-life examples, answers to frequently asked questions, and helpful tables and charts, Harvard University researcher and practitioner Timothy Wilens explains which medications may be prescribed for children and why.

For Adults Who Have ADHD

Barkley, Russell A., Ph.D. *Attention-Deficit Hyperactivity Disorder: A*

Handbook for Diagnosis and Treatment. 4th ed. New York: Guilford Press, 2014.

Barkley, Russell A., Ph.D., and C. M. Benton. *Taking Charge of Adult ADHD*. New York: Guilford Press, 2010.

Hallowell, Edward M., M.D., and Sue Hallowell, LICSW, with Melissa Orlov. *Married to Distraction: How to Restore Intimacy and Strengthen Your Partnership in an Age of Interruption*. New York: Ballantine, 2010.

Hartmann, Thom. *Attention Deficit Disorder: A Different Perception*. Nevada City, CA: Underwood Books, 1997. Thom Hartmann explains some of the positive characteristics sometimes associated with ADHD and provides an explanation of the disorder that can help adults at home, at work, and in school.

Kelly, Kate, and Peggy Ramundo. *You Mean I'm Not Lazy, Stupid, or Crazy?! A Self-Help Book for Adults with Attention Deficit Disorder*. New York: Scribner, 1996.

Kolberg, Judith, and Kathleen Nadeau, Ph.D. *ADD-Friendly Ways to Organize Your Life*. East Sussex, UK: Brunner-Routledge, 2002. This collaboration brings together the best understanding of the disorder with the most effective and practical remedies from ADHD experts in two important fields: professional organization and clinical psychology.

Novotni, Michele, Ph.D. *What Does Everybody Else Know That I Don't? Social Skills Help for Adults with Attention Deficit/Hyperactivity Disorder (AD/HD)*. Forest Lake, MN: Specialty Press, 1999. Social skills help for ADHD adults.

Solden, Sari, M.S., LMFT. *Women with Attention Deficit Disorder*. 2nd ed. Ann Arbor: Introspect Press, 2012. Sari Solden combines real-life histories, treatment experiences, and recent clinical research to highlight the special challenges facing women with attention deficit disorder.

———. *Journeys Through ADDulthood*. London: Walker, 2002. Offers a wealth of wisdom, sound advice, reassuring experiences, and hope for adults with ADHD.

General Books on ADHD

Brown, T. E. *Attention Deficit Disorder: The Unfocused Mind in Children and*

Adults. New Haven: Yale University Press, 2005.

———. *Smart but Stuck: Emotions in Teens and Adults with ADHD.* Hoboken, NJ: Jossey-Bass/Wiley, 2014.

Corman, C. A., and Edward M. Hallowell, M.D. *Positively ADD: Real Success Stories to Inspire Your Dreams.* London: Walker, 2006.

Dawson, P., and R. Guare. *Smart but Scattered: The Revolutionary "Executive Skills" to Helping Kids Reach Their Potential.* New York: Guilford Press, 2009.

Dendy, Chris A. Zeigler. *Teenagers with ADD: A Parents' Guide.* Bethesda, MD: Woodbine House, 1995.

Gallagher, R., H. B. Abikoff, and E. G. Spira. *Organizational Skills Training for Children with ADHD: An Empirically Supported Treatment.* New York: Guilford Press, 2014.

Hallowell, Edward M., M.D., and John J. Ratey, M.D. *Driven to Distraction: Recognizing and Coping with Attention Deficit Disorder from Childhood Through Adulthood.* New York: Pantheon, 1994.

———. *Answers to Distraction.* New York: Bantam, 1996.

———. *Delivered from Distraction.* New York: Ballantine, 2005.

Hinshaw, S. P., and K. Ellison. *ADHD: What Everyone Needs to Know.* New York: Oxford University Press, 2015.

Hinshaw, S. P., and R. M. Scheffler. *The ADHD Explosion: Myths, Medication, Money, and Today's Push for Performance.* New York: Oxford University Press, 2014.

Jensen, Peter S., M.D., and James R. Cooper, M.D., eds. *Attention Deficit Hyperactivity Disorder: State of the Science, Best Practices.* Kingston, NJ: Civic Research Institute, 2002. This is the most comprehensive, authoritative academic volume on the topic available today. Jensen and Cooper bring together various points of view in this superb reference book.

Kaufman, C. *Executive Function in the Classroom.* Baltimore: Brookes Publishing, 2010.

Kohlberg, J., and K. Nadeau. *ADD-Friendly Ways to Organize Your Life.* East Sussex, UK: Brunner-Routledge, 2002.

Lavoie, Richard. *It's So Much Work to Be Your Friend: Helping the Child with Learning Disabilities Find Social Success.* New York: Touchstone, 2006.

Lovecky, D. *Different Minds: Gifted Children with ADHD, Asperger's Syndrome, and Other Learning Deficits.* London: Jessica Kingsley, 2004.

Matlen, Terry. *The Queen of Distraction: How Women with ADHD Can Conquer Chaos, Find Focus, and Get More Done.* Oakland, CA: New Harbinger, 2014.

Nadeau, K., and P. Quinn, eds. *Understanding Women with ADHD.* San Diego: Advantage Books, 2002.

Orlov, Melissa. *The ADHD Effect on Marriage.* Boca Raton, FL: Specialty Press/ADD WareHouse, 2010.

Quinn, P. *Coaching.* San Diego: Advantage Books, 2000.

Ratey, John J., M.D., and Eric Hagerman. *Spark: The Revolutionary New Science of Exercise and the Brain.* Boston: Little, Brown, 2008.

Richardson, W. *The Link Between ADD and Addiction.* Seattle: Piñon Press, 1997.

Rief, S. F. *How to Reach and Teach Children with ADD/ADHD.* 2nd ed. Hoboken, NJ: Jossey-Bass, 2005.

Schultz, J. *Nowhere to Hide: Why Kids with ADHD and LD Hate School and What to Do About It.* Hoboken, NJ: Jossey-Bass, 2011.

Sleeper-Triplett, J. *Empowering Youth with ADHD: Your Guide to Coaching Adolescents and Young Adults, for Coaches, Parents, and Professionals.* Forest Lake, MN: Specialty Press, 2010.

Solden, Sari, M.S., LMFT. *Women with Attention Deficit Disorder.* 2nd ed. Ann Arbor: Introspect Press, 2012.

Surman, C., and T. Bilkey. *Fast Minds: How to Thrive If You Have ADHD (or Think You Might).* New York: Berkley Books, 2014.

Tuckman, A. *More Attention, Less Deficit: Success Stories for Adults with ADHD.* Boca Raton, FL: Specialty Press, 2009.

Vail, Priscilla. *Smart Kids with School Problems: Things to Know and Ways to Help.* New York: Plume, 1989. The late Priscilla Vail, a true pioneer and an exceptional woman, introduced me to the world of learning differences. This book is a classic, along with one of her other books, *Emotion: The*

On-Off Switch for Learning.

Wilens, Timothy E., M.D. *Straight Talk About Psychiatric Medications for Kids.* 4th ed. New York: Guilford Press, 2016.

STATE-BY-STATE SUPPORT AND EDUCATION GROUPS

What follows is a rundown of recommended support and education groups organized by state, and within each state (where applicable) by city. You may notice that there are some states for which there is nothing listed. This is *not* to suggest that you are on your own in those states. Not at all! Rather, when we have not listed a state, it is because we were not able to confirm the contact information by the time this book went to press. That said, please note that the terrific national organization CHADD has branches in every state. Where we have worked with or been in close contact with a CHADD local branch, we have listed that branch within this state listing. But you can go to the CHADD website at www.chadd.org or call their national information line at 800-233-4050 to get the specifics of contact information where you live.

Arizona
Scottsdale

ATTENTION DEFICIT DISORDER CLINIC
www.add-clinic.com
480-424-7200

Tucson

CHADD OF TUCSON (ADULT AND PARENT SUPPORT GROUPS)
www.chaddoftucson.com/chadd-of-tucson/
520-327-7002

Arkansas
Jonesboro

FOCUS, INC.
www.focusinc.org
870-935-2750

Focus targets individuals with developmental disabilities, particularly those who are underserved, either because of the severity of the disability or because of the lack of family and community support.

California

Alameda, Butte, Contra Costa, Humboldt, Lake, Marin, Mendocino, Monterey, Napa, Nevada, Sacramento, San Benito, San Francisco, San Joaquin, San Mateo, Santa Clara, Santa Cruz, Sonoma, and Yolo counties

CHADD OF NORTHERN CALIFORNIA

www.chaddnorcal.org

Palo Alto

HALLOWELL TODARO CENTER

www.hallowelltodaro.com

650-446-4900

San Diego

LEARNING DEVELOPMENT SERVICES

www.learningdevelopmentservices.com

858-581-5050

Email: learndev@aol.com

Providing services for adults, parents, and children.

San Francisco

HALLOWELL CENTER

www.drhallowell.com/san-francisco/

415-967-0061

Colorado
Castle Rock

INSPIRE THE FAMILY

303-229-3348

Email: inspirethefamily@gmail.com

Connecticut

Niantic

CONNECTICUT PARENT ADVOCACY CENTER (STATEWIDE ADVOCACY AND SUPPORT)

www.cpacinc.org

860-739-3089, 800-445-2722

Email: cpac@cpacinc.org

Parents and professionals are welcome to visit CPAC; however, consultants are not available at all times. In order to be sure that there is someone who can assist you, we suggest that you make an appointment or call ahead.

Georgia
Atlanta

ATLANTA SATELLITE OF CHADD (ADULTS, WOMEN WITH ADHD, AND PARENT GROUPS)

www.chadd.net/chapter/193

404-502-5358

Email: atlanta-area@chadd.net

Hawaii
Honolulu

LD-ADHD CENTER OF HAWAII

www.ldcenterofhawaii.com

808-955-4775

Email: contact@ldcenterofhawaii.com

Idaho
Boise

IDAHO PARENTS UNLIMITED, INC. (SUPPORT, INFORMATION, AND ASSISTANCE TO FAMILIES)

www.ipulidaho.org

208-342-5884

Email: parents@ipulidaho.org

Illinois

Chicago

ADHD CENTERS—PETER JAKSA, PH.D.

www.addcenters.com

312-372-4824

Email: drjaksa@addcenters.com

CHICAGO NORTH SHORE ADHD SUPPORT GROUP (CHADD)

www.nsadhd.org

Indiana
Fort Wayne

ALLEN COUNTY CHADD (ADULTS WITH ADHD SUPPORT GROUP)

www.chadd.net/487

260-436-2556

Email: allen-county@chadd.net

Iowa
Des Moines

ASK RESOURCE CENTER (RESOURCE FOR CHILDREN AND ADULTS WITH DISABILITIES)

www.askresource.org

515-243-1713, 800-450-8667

Email: info@askresource.org

Kansas

FAMILIES TOGETHER, INC. (FAMILY INFORMATION NETWORK)

www.familiestogetherinc.org

Garden City: 620-276-6364; Email: gardencity@familiestogetherinc.org

Topeka: 785-233-4777; Email: topeka@familiestogetherinc.org

Wichita: 316-945-7747; Email wichita@familiestogetherinc.org

Kentucky

NEXT STEP 4 ADHD

www.nextstep4adhd.com

Louisville: 502-907-5908

Lexington: 859-609-0520

Offers access to the highest-quality care and resources coupled with the ease and convenience of receiving exceptional care for you and your family in one location.

Louisiana
Metairie

THE CENTER FOR DEVELOPMENT AND LEARNING (CDL)

www.cdl.org

504-840-9786

Email: learn@cdl.org

Provides tools for improving teaching and increasing learning.

New Orleans

FAMILIES HELPING FAMILIES OF SOUTHEAST LOUISIANA

www.fhfsela.org

877-243-7352, 504-943-0343

Provides resources and programming for people with disabilities and their families.

Maine
Farmingdale

MAINE PARENT FEDERATION

www.mpf.org

207-588-1933, 800-870-7746

Provides advocacy, education, and training.

Maryland
Easton

THE LEARNING CONNECTIONS LLC

www.thelearningconnections.net

Beverly Rohman, Learning Consultant and ADHD Coach

410-829-9561

Email: beverlyrohman@gmail.com

Germantown

CLARKE COACHING

www.clarkecoaching.com

301-956-0900

Email: sherry@ClarkeCoaching.com

Silver Spring and Rockville

ADULT ADHD CENTER OF WASHINGTON

www.adultadhdcenterdc.com

202-232-3766

Email: adultADHDcenter@gmail.com

Psychologists and social workers who specialize in ADHD and also do general psychotherapy.

Massachusetts
Sudbury

HALLOWELL CENTER BOSTON METROWEST

www.drhallowellsudbury.com

978-287-0819

Michigan
Ann Arbor

WASHTENAW COUNTY CHADD

www.chadd.net/chapter/355

Email: lwoodcock-burroughs@cnld.org

Support groups for adults with ADHD and parents of children with ADHD.
Birmingham

CHADD OF EASTERN OAKLAND COUNTY

www.chadd.net/chapter/527

248-988-6716

Email: eastern-oakland@chadd.net

Grand Rapids

GRAND RAPIDS OF CHADD

www.chaddgr.org

Missouri
St. Peters

MPACT PARENT TRAINING AND INFORMATION

www.missouriparentsact.org

800-743-7634

Email: info@missouriparentsact.org

Montana
Billings

PARENTS, LET'S UNITE FOR KIDS—PLUK (STATEWIDE INFORMATION, SUPPORT, TRAINING)

www.mtpluk.org

406-255-0540, 800-222-7585

Email: info@mtpluk.org

Nebraska

PTI NEBRASKA (STATEWIDE TRAINING AND INFORMATION FOR FAMILIES WITH SPECIAL NEEDS)

www.pti-nebraska.org

402-346-0525, 800-284-8520

Email: reception@pti-nebraska.org

Nevada
Las Vegas

NEVADA PEP (EDUCATING AND EMPOWERING FAMILIES)

www.nvpep.org/

702-388-8899, 800-216-5188

Email: pepinfo@nvpep.org

New Jersey
Long Beach

ADD ADULT SUPPORT GROUP (ADULTS AND THEIR SIGNIFICANT OTHERS)

www.drlopresti.com/adhd-support-group

732-842-4553

New York
Manhattan

HALLOWELL CENTER NEW YORK

www.hallowellcenter.org

212-799-7777

Email: info@hallowellcenter.org

MANHATTAN ADULT ADD SUPPORT GROUP

www.maaddsg.org

Contact form on website.

THE ADD RESOURCE CENTER

www.addrc.org

646-295-8080

Nassau County

CHADD OF NASSAU COUNTY

www.chadd.net/chapter/105

516-242-3263

Email: nassau-county@chadd.net

North Carolina
Charlotte

MECKLENBURG COUNTY CHADD

www.chadd.net/chapter/355
Email: lwoodcock-burroughs@cnld.org

Ohio
Central Ohio

CHADD OF COLUMBUS
www.columbuschadd.weebly.com
Email: columbus-ohio@chadd.net

Pennsylvania
Pittsburgh

CHADD OF PITTSBURGH
www.pittsburghadd.org/
Contact form on website.
Support group for adults with ADHD.
Pittsburgh Area

CHADD #477
www.chadd.net/chapter/477
412-682-6282
Email: lesliestonepgh@gmail.com

Rhode Island
Riverside

LIFESPAN, BRADLEY HOSPITAL
ADHD Adult Support Group
401-782-4286
Email: info@riaddults.org

South Dakota
Sioux Falls

SOUTH DAKOTA PARENT CONNECTION (SDPC)
www.sdparent.org

605-361-3171, 800-640-4553

Email: sdpc@sdparent.org

Connecting families of children with special needs with training, information, and resources.

Virginia
Virginia Beach

HR CHADD

www.meetup.com/HRCHADD/

Washington
Kirkland

HALLOWELL TODARO ADHD CENTER

www.hallowelltodaro.com

425-999-4227

Email: info@hallowelltodaro.com

Seattle

HALLOWELL TODARO ADHD CENTER

www.hallowelltodaro.com

206-420-7345

Email: info@hallowelltodaro.com

Washington, D.C.

ADVOCATES FOR JUSTICE AND EDUCATION (EDUCATION AND SUPPORT)

www.aje-dc.org

202-678-8060, 888-327-8060

Wyoming
Buffalo

PARENT INFORMATION CENTER (PARENTS HELPING PARENTS OF WYOMING, INC.)

www.wpic.org

307-684-2277, 800-660-9742

Email: info@wpic.org

Canada
Vancouver, British Columbia

VANCOUVER ADULT ADD SUPPORT GROUP

www.addcoach4u.com/canadianadhdsupportgroups.html

604-263-6993

Email: pete@addcoach4u.com

Meet other adults with ADHD and share support and encouragement.

Select Bibliography

Introduction

Barkley, Russell A., Ph.D. "Reduced Life Expectancy in ADHD." Interview. *Carlat Child Psychiatry Report,* January 2020.

Chapter 1: A Spectrum of Traits

Barkley, Russell A., Ph.D. *Taking Charge of ADHD: The Complete, Authoritative Guide for Parents.* 4th ed. New York: Guilford Press, 2020. (A classic from the man who, more than anyone else, established ADHD as a real, biologically based, heritable condition.)

———. *When an Adult You Love Has ADHD: Professional Advice for Parents, Partners, and Siblings.* Washington, DC: American Psychological Association Press, 2016.

Hedden, T., and J.D.E. Gabrieli. "The Ebb and Flow of Attention in the Human Brain." *Nature Neuroscience* 2006;9 863–65. https://www.nature.com/articles/nn0706-863.

Jackson, Maggie. *Distracted: Reclaiming Our Focus in a World of Lost Attention.* Amherst, NY: Prometheus Books, 2018.

Matlen, Terry. *The Queen of Distraction: How Women with ADHD Can Conquer Chaos, Find Focus, and Get More Done.* Oakland, CA: New Harbinger, 2014.

Poole, Jim, M.D., FAAP. *Flipping ADHD on Its Head: How to Turn Your Child's "Disability" into Their Greatest Strength.* Austin, TX: Greenleaf Book Group Press, 2020.

Solden, Sari, M.S., LMFT. *Women with Attention Deficit Disorder.* 2nd ed. Ann Arbor: Introspect Press, 2012.

Spiegelhalter, David. *The Art of Statistics: How to Learn from Data.* New York: Basic Books, 2019.

Vail, Priscilla L. *Smart Kids with School Problems: Things to Know and Ways to Help.* New York: Plume, 1989. (An all-time classic.)

Chapter 2: Understanding the Demon of the Mind

Boyatzis, R. E., K. Rochford, and A. I. Jack. "Antagonistic Neural Networks Underlying Differentiated Leadership Roles." *Frontiers in Human Neuroscience* 2014 Mar 4;8:114. https://www.frontiersin.org/articles/10.3389/fnhum.2014.00114/full.

Chai, X. J., N. Ofen, J.D.E. Gabrieli, and S. Whitfield-Gabrieli. "Selective Development of Anticorrelated Networks in the Intrinsic Functional Organization of the Human Brain." *Journal of Cognitive Neuroscience* 2014 Mar;26(3):501–13. https://pubmed.ncbi.nlm.nih.gov/23812094/.

———. "Development of Deactivation of the Default-Mode Network During Episodic Memory Formation." *NeuroImage* 2014 Jan 1;84:932–38. https://pubmed.ncbi.nlm.nih.gov/24064072/.

Kumar, J., S. J. Iwabuchi, B. A. Völlm, and L. Palaniyappan. "Oxytocin Modulates the Effective Connectivity Between the Precuneus and the Dorsolateral Prefrontal Cortex." *European Archives of Psychiatry and Clinical Neuroscience* 2019 Feb 7. https://link.springer.com/article/10.1007/s00406-019-00989-z.

Mattfeld, A. T., J.D.E. Gabrieli, J. Biederman, T. Spencer, A. Brown, A. Kotte, E. Kagan, and S. Whitfield-Gabrieli. "Brain Differences Between Persistent and Remitted Attention-Deficit/Hyperactivity Disorder." *Brain* 2014 Sep;137(Pt 9):2423–28. https://pubmed.ncbi.nlm.nih.gov/24916335/.

Raichle, Marcus. "The Brain's Default Mode Network." *Annual Review of Neuroscience* 2015 July;38:433–47. https://www.annualreviews.org/doi/10.1146/annurev-neuro-071013-014030.

Tryon, Warren. *Cognitive Neuroscience and Psychology: Network Principles for a Unified Theory.* Cambridge, MA: Academic Press, 2014.

Chapter 3: The Cerebellum Connection

Chevalier, N., V. Parent, M. Rouillard, F. Simard, M. C. Guay, and C. Verret. "The Impact of a Motor-Cognitive Remediation Program on Attentional Functions of Preschoolers with ADHD Symptoms." *Journal of Attention Disord*ers 2017 Nov;21(13):1121–29. http://journals.sagepub.com/doi/abs/10.1177/1087054712468485.

Guell, X., J.D.E. Gabrieli, and J. D. Schmahmann. "Embodied Cognition and the Cerebellum: Perspectives from the Dysmetria of Thought and the Universal Cerebellar Transform Theories." *Cortex* 2018 Mar; 100:140–48. https://pubmed.ncbi.nlm.nih.gov/28779872/.

Schmahmann, Jeremy D. "The Cerebellum and Cognition." *Neuroscience Letters* 2019 Jan 1;688:62–75. https://neuro.psychiatryonline.org/doi/full/10.1176/jnp.16.3.367.

———. "Disorders of the Cerebellum: Ataxia, Dysmetria of Thought, and the Cerebellar Cognitive Affective Syndrome." *Journal of Neuropsychiatry and Clinical Neurosciences* 2004;16(3):367–78. https://neuro.psychiatryonline.org/doi/full/10.1176/jnp.16.3.367.

———, J. B. Weilburg, and J. C. Sherman. "The Neuropsychiatry of the Cerebellum—Insights from the Clinic." *Cerebellum* 2007;6(3):254–67. https://link.springer.com/article/10.1080%2F14734220701490995.

Chapter 4: The Healing Power of Connection

The Adverse Childhood Experiences Study. https://acestoohigh.com/2012/10/03/the-adverse-childhood-experiences-study-the-largest-most-important-public-health-study-you-never-heard-of-began-in-an-obesity-clinic/.

Christakis, Nicholas A., M.D., Ph.D., and James H. Fowler, Ph.D. *Connected: How Your Friends' Friends' Friends Affect Everything You Feel, Think, and Do.* Boston: Little, Brown, 2009.

Harding, Kelli. *The Rabbit Effect: Live Longer, Healthier, and Happier with the Groundbreaking Science of Kindness.* New York: Atria Books, 2019.

"How Family Dinners Improve Students' Grades." https://www.ectutoring.com/resources/articles/family-dinners-improve-students-grades.

Kumar, J., S. J. Iwabuchi, B. A. Völlm, and L. Palaniyappan. "Oxytocin Modulates the Effective Connectivity Between the Precuneus and the Dorsolateral Prefrontal Cortex." *European Archives of Psychiatry and Clinical Neuroscience* 2019 Feb 7. https://link.springer.com/article/10.1007/s00406-019-00989-z.

Lieberman, Matthew D. *Social: Why Our Brains Are Wired to Connect.* New York: Broadway Books, 2014.

Murthy, Vivek H., M.D. *Together: The Healing Power of Connection in a Sometimes Lonely World.* New York: Harper Wave, 2020.

Rowe, John Wallis, M.D., and Robert L. Kahn, Ph.D. *Successful Aging.* New York: Pantheon, 1998.

Vaillant, George. *Triumphs of Experience: The Men of the Harvard Grant Study.* Cambridge, MA: Belknap Press of Harvard University Press, 2015.

Chapter 5: Find Your Right Difficult

Bloom, Benjamin S. *Developing Talent in Young People.* New York: Ballantine, 1985. (A classic.)

Brooks, David. *The Road to Character.* New York: Random House, 2015.

Hallowell, Edward M., M.D. *Shine: Using Brain Science to Get the Best from Your People.* Cambridge, MA: Harvard Business Review Press, 2011.

Kolbe, Kathy. *Conative Connection: Uncovering the Link Between Who You Are and How You Perform.* Phoenix, AZ: Kolbe Corporation, 1997.

Chapter 6: Create Stellar Environments

Campbell, T. Colin, and Thomas M. Campbell II. *The China Study: Revised and Expanded Edition: The Most Comprehensive Study of Nutrition Ever Conducted and the Startling Implications for Diet, Weight Loss, and Long-Term Health.* Dallas, TX: BenBella Books, 2016.

Frates, Beth, M.D., et al. *The Lifestyle Medicine Handbook: An Introduction to the Power of Healthy Habits.* Monterey, CA: Healthy Learning, 2018.

Maguire, Caroline, PCC, M.Ed. *Why Will No One Play with Me? The Play Better Plan to Help Children of All Ages Make Friends and Thrive.* New York: Grand Central Publishing, 2019.

Vaillant, George E., M.D. *Aging Well: Surprising Guideposts to a Happier Life from the Landmark Harvard Study of Adult Development.* Boston: Little, Brown, 2003.

Chapter 7: Move to Focus, Move to Motivate: The Power of Exercise

Brewer, J. A., P. D. Worhunsky, J. R. Gray, Y. Y. Tang, J. Weber, and H. Kober. "Meditation Experience Is Associated with Differences in Default Mode Network Activity and Connectivity." *Proceedings of the National Academy of Sciences of the United States of America* 2011 Dec 13;108(50):20254–59. https://pubmed.ncbi.nlm.nih.gov/22114193/.

Chevalier, N., V. Parent, M. Rouillard, F. Simard, M. C. Guay, and C. Verret. "The Impact of a Motor-Cognitive Remediation Program on Attentional Functions of Preschoolers with ADHD Symptoms." *Journal of Attention Disorders* 2017 Nov;21(13):1121–29. http://journals.sagepub.com/doi/abs/10.1177/1087054712468485.

Chou, C. C., and C. J. Huang. "Effects of an 8-Week Yoga Program on Sustained Attention and Discrimination Function in Children with Attention Deficit Hyperactivity Disorder." *PeerJ* 2017 Jan 12;5:e2883. https://pubmed.ncbi.nlm.nih.gov/28097075/.

Hölzel, B. K., J. Carmody, M. Vangel, C. Congleton, S. M. Yerramsetti, T. Gard, and S. W. Lazar. "Mindfulness Practice Leads to Increases in Regional Brain Gray Matter Density." *Psychiatry Research* 2011 Jan 30;191(1):36–43. https://pubmed.ncbi.nlm.nih.gov/21071182/.

Levin, K. "The Dance of Attention: Toward an Aesthetic Dimension of Attention-Deficit." *Integrative Psychological and Behavioral Science* 2018 Mar;52(1):129–51. https://link.springer.com/article/10.1007%2Fs12124-017-9413-7.

Mailey, E. L., D. Dlugonski, W. W. Hsu, and M. Segar. "Goals Matter: Exercising for Well-Being but Not Health or Appearance Predicts Future Exercise Among Parents." *Journal of Physical Activity and Health* 2018 Nov 1;15(11):857–65. https://journals.humankinetics.com/view/journals/jpah/15/11/article-p857.xml.

Ratey, John J., M.D., and Eric Hagerman. *Spark: The Revolutionary New Science of Exercise and the Brain.* Boston: Little, Brown, 2008.

Suarez-Manzano, S., A. Ruiz-Ariza, M. De la Torre-Cruz, and E. J. Martínez-López. "Acute and Chronic Effect of Physical Activity on Cognition and

Behaviour in Young People with ADHD: A Systematic Review of Intervention Studies." *Research in Developmental Disabilities* 2018 Jun;77:12–23. https://pubmed.ncbi.nlm.nih.gov/29625261/.

Chapter 8: Medication: The Most Powerful Tool Everyone Fears

Alexander, Bruce K. *The Globalization of Addiction: A Study in Poverty of the Spirit.* New York: Oxford University Press, 2008.

Biederman, J., M. C. Monuteaux, T. Spencer, T. E. Wilens, H. A. Macpherson, and S. V. Faraone. "Stimulant Therapy and Risk for Subsequent Substance Use Disorders in Male Adults with ADHD: A Naturalistic Controlled 10-Year Follow-Up Study." *American Journal of Psychiatry* 2008;165:597–603. https://ajp.psychiatryonline.org/doi/10.1176/appi.ajp.2007.07091486.

Cortese, S., et al. "Comparative Efficacy and Tolerability of Medications for Attention-Deficit Hyperactivity Disorder in Children, Adolescents, and Adults: A Systematic Review and Network Meta-Analysis." *Psychiatry* 2018 Sep;5(9):727–38. https://www.thelancet.com/journals/lanpsy/article/PIIS2215-0366(18)30269-4/fulltext.

Fay, T. B., and M. A. Alpert. "Cardiovascular Effects of Drugs Used to Treat Attention-Deficit/Hyperactivity Disorder, Part 2: Impact on Cardiovascular Events and Recommendations for Evaluation and Monitoring." *Cardiology in Review* 2019 Jul/Aug;27(4):173–78. https://pubmed.ncbi.nlm.nih.gov/30531411/.

Foote, Jeffrey, Ph.D., Carrie Wilkens, Ph.D., and Nicole Kosanke, Ph.D. *Beyond Addiction: How Science and Kindness Help People.* New York: Scribner, 2014.

Kolar, D., A. Keller, M. Golfinopoulos, L. Cumyn, C. Syer, and L. Hechtman. "Treatment of Adults with Attention-Deficit/Hyperactivity Disorder." *Neuropsychiatric Disease and Treatment* 2008 Feb;4(1):107–21. https://pubmed.ncbi.nlm.nih.gov/18728745/.

Pollan, Michael. *How to Change Your Mind.* New York: Penguin Press, 2018.

Sederer, Lloyd. *The Addiction Solution.* New York: Scribner, 2019.

Shaw, M., P. Hodgkins, H. Caci, S. Young, J. Kahle, A. G. Woods, and L. E. Arnold. "A Systematic Review and Analysis of Long-Term Outcomes in Attention Deficit Hyperactivity Disorder: Effects of Treatment and Non-

Treatment." *BMC Medicine* 2012 Sep 4;10:99. https://bmcmedicine.biomedcentral.com/articles/10.1186/1741-7015-10-99.

Szalavitz, Maia. *Unbroken Brain: A Revolutionary New Way of Understanding Addiction*. New York: Picador, 2017.

Westbrook, A., R. van den Bosch, J. I. Määttä, L. Hofmans, D. Papadopetraki, R. Cools, and M. J. Frank. "Dopamine Promotes Cognitive Effort by Biasing the Benefits Versus Costs of Cognitive Work." *Science* 2020 Mar 20;367(6484):1362–66. https://science.sciencemag.org/content/367/6484/1362.

Wilens, Timothy E., M.D. *Straight Talk About Psychiatric Medications for Kids*. 4th ed. New York: Guilford Press, 2016.